W9-DEA-336

Real Kids

Real Kids

Creating Meaning in Everyday Life

Susan Engel

Harvard University Press · Cambridge, Massachusetts · London, England · 2005

Printed in the United States of America

Library of Congress Cataloging-in-Publication Data

Engel, Susan L.
Real Kids : Creating Meaning in Everyday Life / Susan Engel.
p. cm.
Includes bibliographical references (p.) and index.
ISBN 0-674-01883-4 (alk. paper)
1. Cognition in children. I. Title.

BF723.C5E49 2005
115.4′13–dc22 2005046005

FOR MARGERY B. FRANKLIN

Contents

Preface *ix*

Introduction 1

1 What We See and What We Miss 6

2 A Glance Backward: What Have We Learned about Children? 44

3 Spheres of Reality in Childhood 92

4 Toward a More Complete Understanding of Children 136

5 Why This Matters, and to Whom 174

Notes *197*

Index *211*

Preface

This book begins and ends with my intense curiosity about the way young children think and behave, and my sense that there are untapped riches to be found in the close observation of children as they play, talk, argue, and explore—in short, as they confront themselves and the world around them. Throughout my years as a researcher, again and again I have found that some unexpected moment of a child's behavior offered important clues about how children think and what they think about. The great psychologist Henry James said that often it was a fleeting gesture or a glance between two people at a dinner party that set him on the path of a new narrative—these unexpected moments provided "the vital particle" that would spark years of thought and work. So too can three minutes of a child playing with a stick, struggling over a toy with a peer, or asking a series of questions to a parent provide the curious, open-minded researcher with the vital particle for new research and new insight. While gathering my thoughts in preparation for writing this book, I came upon a wonderful description by Dennie Wolf of a little girl at play with her mother. The two were setting up some small wooden toys representing trees and animals to create a jungle scene. The toy giraffes kept falling over, which presented a problem to the little girl as she tried to arrange things to her liking. Finally, she pushed some toy shrubs up against the baby giraffe to hold it standing up, and said to her mother, "Pretend it was called the messy jungle." The minute I read this description, I realized I had found a vital particle to the story I wanted to tell about the way in which children construct and explore their worlds.

Children are enormously creative at using gestures, objects, and words to construct and express versions of the world as they experience it. Their zeal for such creativity is matched only by the energy with which they want to make sense of their daily experiences. But often their creativity and sense-making efforts are enmeshed with one another. In addition, the four-year-old child's "sense" may be quite different from adult "sense." Clearly the little girl's original intent was to have something other than a messy jungle—perhaps a neat jungle, or something altogether different (a zoo, a farm, a family?). In the end, however, the limitations of her toys led her to announce a compromise: a messy jungle. This small passage captures two themes that are central to my argument: First, the child's meanings, or construals, as well as her intentions, must be interpreted from her own perspective—we cannot assume that the world looks to the child as it does to adults. And second, the very idea of a "messy jungle" evokes some of what has been lost in our efforts to find order and pattern in the child's thinking. While I am as eager as any other psychologist to understand how children think, what they feel, and what the world looks like to them, I am reluctant to do so by imposing scientific neatness, adult logic, or conventional order on the way they think, if in so doing I miss the real nature of the phenomena. There is good reason to believe that there is as much messy jungle as there is garden in the mind of the young child.

I have found that there are two kinds of developmental researchers—those who know a great deal about research, and those who know a great deal about children. My wish is that more of us would come to know about both, and put those two sorts of knowledge in relation to one another. This book is an attempt to move myself and others closer to such integration.

In writing this book I depended heavily on the ideas, feedback, arguments, support, and inspiration of others. First I want to thank my editor at Harvard, Elizabeth Knoll, whose eagerness about this topic and thoughtful comments on the manuscript were vitally important to the process and to the book itself. I also want to thank Julie Carlson, who made the final phase of this project an unexpected pleasure, and whose editing greatly improved my writing.

I wish to thank all the teachers, parents, and children who allowed me to observe and record them in their everyday lives. In addition, there were many scholars who helped me during the development of this book, and although many of them might disagree vehemently with its contents, I am immensely grateful to them all. Paul Harris's love of ideas is matched only by his love of data. He is a daunting critic, and a generous and delightful colleague. I also thank Robert Kavanaugh—I depend on him in countless ways, and savor every one of our discussions about developmental psychology. I thank Liz Bertsch, Katherine Bouton, Jerome Bruner, Carol Feldman, Marcelle Langendal, Saskia Larraz, Scottie Mills, Katherine Nelson, and Marlene Sandstrom for our many conversations about children and science. Kathy Engel and Tinka Topping, as always, offered ideas, suggestions, questions, and tremendous support along the way. Justine and Ella provided me, once again, with wonderful stories. Feedback from the Austen-Riggs/Williams study group was helpful to me in clarifying some of my arguments.

Several people read the manuscript and offered me generous and invaluable feedback: Herman Engel, Mary Gauvain, Betty Prashker, and Christie Schueler, as well as two anonymous readers.

My sons Jake, Will, and Sam, and my husband, Tom Levin, continue to be the lights of my life, as well as wonderful sources of ideas and inspiration. Jenno Topping provided support in so many ways I cannot even list them all, ranging from critical readings of the manuscript to rich descriptions of her two young children, as well as constant encouragement and problem solving of every kind.

It is rare in life that one's teacher becomes one's best friend, and yet remains a teacher in the best sense of the word. I am lucky enough to have such a friend and teacher, Margery B. Franklin. She was my first psychology professor in college, and continues to be the most interesting person I know with whom to talk about the minds of young children. Many of the ideas in this book began in the conversations and questions she and I have been mulling over for twenty-seven years.

Real Kids

Introduction

I was a teacher of young children before I was a psychologist. Perhaps that is why, ever since I began reading research in developmental psychology in college, I have had a nagging sense that something was amiss. The children depicted in the studies I read were not like the children I encountered in everyday life. For every study that identified something about children invisible to the naked eye, there was an experiment that seemed to render the child into something less than what she really was. For every useful pattern or predictable response elicited through experiments, there was some behavior or quality I had seen with my own two eyes that was absent from the view conveyed by research.

As I began to do research of my own, primarily focusing on narrative development, I found that children's stories, particularly those told by children younger than age seven, offered glimpses of a complex inner life not captured by the predominant theories about young children. Often those things that researchers, including myself, could quantify—such as when a certain task, like grouping blocks, was generally mastered, or when children know that it is their own face in the mirror—were the least interesting aspects of the children I knew, whereas the most interesting aspects—how children share a make-believe scenario in their play, or develop stories as they are telling them—fit awkwardly into the prevailing analytic methods. As Einstein once said, "Not everything that counts can be counted, and not everything that is counted counts." This seemed frustratingly true of the research on children's stories and children's play. Though many studies and theories in the past seventy years have been profound, accurate, and helpful, taken together they could lead one to a seriously distorted picture of what children are like.

My experience gathering children's stories, watching children play, and perhaps just as valuable, working in many classrooms, has convinced me that the prevailing model of children among researchers is too sanitized. The child in the park, on the bus, or overheard in the grocery store is more complex, more mentally active (but in a distinctively childlike way), and less oriented toward adult tasks than the research suggests. Indeed, often the child implied by the studies bears little resemblance to the children we encounter in everyday settings. But I do think that the real child can be known through research that takes the child's perspective into account and, equally important, studies children in settings familiar to them—settings that allow them to play and talk as they naturally love to do. Furthermore, what we might learn from such research could have important implications not only for our model of development, but also for the way we work with children in schools.

In recent years, as I thought about how our collective image of children needed to change, I began to ask myself when and how psychologists had come to such a sanitized and overly rational view of children's thinking. This led me to try and sum up what psychologists have learned about children in the past century (give or take a decade or two). Had researchers been simply refining Piaget's view of children as little scientists, creating ideas about the world and systematically testing and revising these ideas, or had the basic paradigm shifted—and if so, in what way? While considering this question, it dawned on me that though there had been some powerful challenges to Piagetian theory since his work first emerged, he remained at the center of our collective consciousness regarding development. Overall, the bulk of contemporary psychology concerning itself with children's minds is still, in one way or another, a response to Piaget—researchers agree with him and attempt to extend or flesh out a particular idea, they disagree and attempt to show what he missed or mischaracterized, or they rediscover an early claim of his and pin it down with new research methods. But much of this work is still oriented toward the themes, claims, and questions he set out all those years ago. We all seem still to be in a conversation with him, sometimes adoring, sometimes rebellious, sometimes in the grip of his intellectual authority, and sometimes simply obediently carrying out his agenda. This book addresses two topics. First, what have we learned about children in the past seventy years or so? What model or image of childhood has our research led us to? Answering this question leads to the second topic: the ways in which our image of children has gone awry, and what a fuller, more accurate picture of children might look like.

The book begins, in Chapter 1, by describing some of the unexpected things children do and say that suggest our current model is inaccurate. Although we often find such behavior entertaining and cute, and although contemporary research generally dismisses it as unimportant, these examples hold valuable clues regarding the nature of childhood, and how children make sense of their world. Because theories in developmental psychology are almost impossible to disentangle from the methods used to test them, Chapter 1 also offers a conceptual framework for thinking about how methods of research lead to a certain picture of children.

Chapter 2 takes stock of what Piaget and his descendents have learned over the past seventy years. Though at best it merely captures vast bodies of research in overly brief descriptions (sometimes glossing over career-shaking disagreements), this chapter attempts to summarize what we have learned, and to characterize the most influential ideas and shifts within the field. This chapter is not exhaustive, or even complete. Instead it is meant to give readers an overview of a large, diverse body of research, and in so doing, reveal some of the biases and assumptions of that research. The account given is obviously my interpretation of the field, and conveys my own sense of what the major milestones have been. Having sketched a model of children based on existing research, I argue that the model is askew.

Chapter 3 describes what I think is missing from current research, and proposes a somewhat different view of children. This view emphasizes children's imaginative interpretations of experience as well as highlights the fluctuating nature of children's stance toward the world, which causes these interpretations to shift.

Because I believe that the methods we use for investigating development have played such an important role in shaping what we have learned (and missed), in Chapter 4 I turn to suggestions for ways to study the fluctuating, experiential aspects of childhood outlined in Chapter 3. I also include discussions of bodies of work that either already encompass such a view, or could lead us to greater knowledge about how children experience—and transform—reality.

I hope this book will encourage my fellow researchers to ask new questions of their methods and to consider aspects of the child's experience that they might earlier have dismissed as unimportant or inaccessible to research. But because I have spent my life working directly with children and those who teach children, this book is also meant for classroom teachers—as well as parents, children's first teachers. In Chapter 5, I discuss the implications of a "messier" or more dynamic view of children, one that takes their perspective and inner lives into account. This chapter outlines some specific suggestions that follow from considering the dynamic and rich inner lives of young children.

This book both is, and is not, "developmental." It is about young children, and how and what they think. It is a review of sorts, of developmental theories and research, and argues for a new approach to thinking about and investigating children. But it is not intended to provide a new theory of development in the sense of outlining specific stages of development, identifying causes or sources of change, or teasing apart influences on developmental outcomes. It may be that scholars who are influenced by what they read here will conduct research that does eventually offer us new data and conclusions about specific developmental changes and sources of outcomes, but this book is only a first step in opening up the way we think about young children's minds.

There are many extended examples in the pages that follow, far more than are typically included in a book by a developmental psychologist. There are two reasons for this. First, I fervently hope teachers and parents will be drawn to this book, and will find that such examples clarify and illustrate the ideas presented. Second and perhaps more important, I implicitly promote the model of the naturalist, who focuses on extended examples of real phenomena in natural settings. Including such examples in this book is my way of practicing what I preach.

What We See and What We Miss

1

Children are not simple, nor are they transparent. Though they live among adults and will become adults, they are not merely incomplete adults. Much of the time, in fact, adults and children do not even seem to inhabit the same mental world. The child's thoughts, preoccupations, and interpretations of the world around him are quite different from those that characterize most adults' ideas about their world.

Most readers, including my fellow psychologists, will probably read the preceding paragraph and nod as if what I have written is obvious or perhaps unimportant. But the ramifications of the difference between the mind of the child and that of the adult are huge. Our research, educational practices, and even parenting wisdom often do not reflect an understanding that children's inner lives are complex and different than the inner lives of adults. Recently the developmental psychologist Barbara Rogoff made the excellent and well-documented point that one of the ways children develop is by absorbing the values, habits, and methods of their culture even when they are not actively participating in an adult task, ritual, or gathering.[1] To illustrate this idea she presented a beautiful photograph of young girls in Mexico. The children, ranging in age from four to eight years old, were sitting on a bench in their rural village, quietly watching as their mothers and older sisters were engaged in weaving, an advanced and complex activity highly valued in their community. Rogoff pointed out that even though the children seemed like passive observers, they were learning a lot about what was going on, about how things are done, how to work, and what is important in their culture. But as I looked at the image, I wondered if the children really were watching the older women weave, and I felt sure that one couldn't assume much about their thoughts.

Rogoff's photograph and her explanation of it reminded me of an experience I had had the previous summer that seemed similar, yet had brought me to a totally different conclusion. I was watching a Little League game in the field behind a small school in my rural Massachusetts hometown. There were all kinds of people at the game on this sunny summer evening—relatives and friends of the Little League players, as well as the players and coaches themselves. There was a lot of activity and many different kinds of conversations going on. Rogoff might have said that the younger children, mostly siblings of the players, milling around on the side of the baseball field, were learning a great deal about the customs, cognitions, and skills of their community by watching their older brothers and sisters play, and by listening to their parents cheer, coach, and talk among themselves. One might have assumed that the younger children, like the girls in Mexico, were soaking up the ways of the older people surrounding them. At some point, however, I stopped watching the game and noticed two preschoolers on the lawn next to me. I saw that they were deeply engaged in a game of "baby puppy," fairly oblivious to the adults and older children around them. One child was crawling on the grass on all fours, barking, while another child stroked his head and pretended to feed him morsels of food. When an adult called out for the puppy child to go get a blanket out of the car, the child turned toward the adult and barked at him. What I saw was not a group of small children watching to see what the adult world was like, but small children constructing a world of their own, one that reflected their inner lives.

Usually examples like the baby puppy story are offered to demonstrate the charm of childhood. Psychologists, parents, and teachers are all likely to smile in delight at the whimsy of children's linguistic creations and moments of original or unconventional behavior.

Most of us notice such gems and are amused, but quickly move on to the more "important" or revealing aspects of the child's behavior. Depending on our perspective (parent, teacher, clinical psychologist, or developmental researcher), we are interested in what children know and can do and how well they are progressing in one way or another. We often see early forms of rationality, purposefulness, and adult organization, sometimes to the exclusion of behavior that seems more foreign or enigmatic to us. Sometimes what we see is the absence of adult qualities, and we fail to see what is there instead. We tend to see children as future adults, rather than seeing them on their own terms.

THE LENSES WE USE

A parent wonders whether his child is smart or morally good, whether her behavior holds clues to what kind of adult she will be, or whether she is more like her brother or her mother. Most clinical psychologists focus on children's social and emotional problems, and are oriented toward working with individual children who have such problems. The clinician thinks about the child's relationship to parents, siblings, teachers, and peers.

Researchers are another kettle of fish. Usually those who study developmental psychology are trained to look for characteristics or behaviors that typify a certain age or stage of development. For instance, a developmental psychologist interested in cognition might compare how five- and ten-year-olds perform a certain task involving blocks or numbers. Such research aims to identify the ways in which the five-year-olds are both like each other and different from all the ten-year-olds on some particular dimension (say, numerical skills or problem solving). Another psychologist, interested in peer relations, might want to know whether socially awkward children in middle childhood respond differently to situations than socially successful children. In that case the goal is to find out the ways in which awkward children are like one another and different from popular children, and to identify the range of situations and behaviors that are affected by their awkwardness (for example, a child's social difficulties might play a role in his response to failure, but might not affect his ability to deal with authority figures). While clinicians think about what is unusual in a child, and how to help that child be more like other children, most researchers are looking for what various groups of children have in common.

As the field of developmental psychology has grown and matured, our questions—as well as our means for answering them—have become more subtle and complex. For instance, where we once asked whether young children believed an object existed even when they couldn't see it, we now ask whether a four-year-old knows that what another person sees is different from what she sees, and that what the other person sees affects what he or she knows about a situation (often referred to in the field as theory-of-mind research). Where we once asked whether children had different temperaments (such as easy or difficult) and looked to identify whether those temperaments stayed with children through school, we now ask whether the mother's specific responses to a child during play can modify or amplify the child's temperament. In other words our questions have become more refined and more ambitious, to match our more sophisticated research methods. Yet one aspect of our research has remained fairly consistent. Researchers often have little direct interaction with the children in their studies (usually because research assistants and students are carrying out the research). When they do, they may only encounter children as subjects—that is, they may only see the children who participate in the study, and only when those children are engaged in the target task. The experimental task and the coding procedures used create a kind of screen between the researcher and the child. In other words, much of researchers' exposure to children happens in highly constrained laboratory settings. Though the clinician and the researcher have different methods and motivations in their work with children, they share the problem of incomplete access to children.

What the clinician, the researcher, and some parents have in common, though for different reasons, is their tendency to miss important behaviors that do not fit whatever psychological framework they are using. Often behaviors such as a spontaneous outburst of lyricism or fantasy slip by the adult altogether. When we developmental psychologists are done marveling at a moment of whimsy or childishness, we most often move on, eager to look for "regular" behavior—attempts to navigate the everyday world, behaviors that show what kinds of problem solving the child uses, or utterances that reveal an inner logic. We watch the way children organize objects and toys to get a picture of what kinds of categories and concepts they use to think. We observe the way they correct their gestures while building with blocks in order to better understand how children modify strategies to fit new experiences in everyday life—for example, when a big block is too heavy on top of a little block, does it change the way the child builds the pile the next time? We record her use of verb tenses to understand how and when she acquires a sense of time and perspective, as well as when she masters the subtle rules of language.

Too often, in our search for tokens of rational thought in children's behavior, we miss the abundant signs of thought that does not conform to conventional, goal-directed logic. I am talking here not of unbalanced or pathological thought, but of what the anthropologist Richard Schweder has called nonrational thought.[2] We look for analogues to our own ways of thinking, and miss the kinds of thinking that have no easy analogue in adult functioning. Often, because our own research foci must be well defined and fairly narrow, we categorize whatever behavior we see as reflecting only one aspect of mental life: we take a given gesture or action to reflect cognitive, social, or emotional processes, and think of the behavior as being either conscious or unconscious. The problem with abiding by these constraints is that they lead to a distorted view of the child's inner life. Not only do we miss important phenomena, but we also misinterpret the phenomena to which we do attend.

In my twenty years of child watching, as a researcher, teacher, and mother, I have rarely seen a child who functions purely rationally or purely irrationally. I have also rarely seen a situation that could be characterized as either completely private or completely social. (For instance, soon after the "baby puppy" barked at the Dad in response to being asked to get a blanket from the car, the Dad said, "Heh. Well if that little puppy don't get over there and get the blanket I'm gonna kick him in the butt"—at which point the boy jumped up and ran over to get the blanket.)

Though not prevalent, the idea that children's thoughts, abilities, and feelings cannot be understood in isolation from one another can be traced back almost one hundred years. In the early part of the twentieth century, the German developmental psychologist Heinz Werner, one of the three great theorists of developmental psychology (along with the Russian Lev Vygotsky and the Swiss Jean Piaget), said about his colleagues in psychology, "The living world of things, in which the human being participates with his feelings, strivings and reflections, does virtually not exist for this psychology [the psychology of objective-technical perception], but only the cold, thinglike, and distanced world of relative closure, which in truth is hardly ever realized."[3] He was arguing against a psychology that isolated behaviors for experimental purposes to such a point that psychologists no longer were considering real people in all their complexity. For developmental psychologists, Werner's criticism of mainstream psychology is particularly relevant. That cold, "thinglike" world Werner spoke of has little to do with the young children one encounters in everyday life, who, like adults, participate in the world with feelings, strivings, and yes, reflections.

Young children are not easy to characterize because, in part, they are messy. By this I do not mean that they spill things or leave their toys lying around. I mean that their behavior is dynamic and often inconsistent, shifting rapidly from one orientation to another. Because they are in such a rapid period of change, their abilities, feelings, motivations, and behaviors are often in transition and hard to characterize in a neat way. Of course adults also shift their attention within brief periods of time, moving from one frame of mind to another. For instance, while attending a tedious meeting an adult might lapse into a daydream about the meal she is going to cook that evening, the argument she had with her spouse earlier that day, or a fantasy about someone sitting opposite in the room. But by and large, adults do this kind of frame switching privately, almost invisibly, and are able to maintain the appearance of steady engagement, as well as some focus on the original task. Dealing with the kinds of dynamic shifts endemic to early childhood is particularly challenging for developmental psychologists who seek patterns in children's behavior and growth, and hope to generalize from small groups of children to the larger population.

Children between the ages of two and seven seem particularly changeable from one moment to the next because the domains of experience that so often neatly contain our adult lives are not yet formed or delineated in the lives of young children. (Researchers such as Elizabeth Spelke and Susan Carey argue that domains of knowledge such as numbers or biology are present and defined early in infancy, but I use the term "domain" here to describe a way of construing experience rather than a body of related knowledge.[4]) The kinds of flow I am referring to here help explain why a child who is hard at work on a task (say cleaning a tabletop, or tracing letters in a book) can, in a second, be drawn into a wild spate of rhyming, spitting, or pretending—a shift that would be hard to comprehend (and might even indicate mental illness) in the behavior of, for instance, a colleague at work. Research, as well as everyday experience, shows us that adults are more likely to constrain their focus, choose a mode of functioning and stick to it, and attend to the demands of a situation as it has been presented to them. Many eighteen-year-olds, for example, can respond to the challenge of taking the SAT by sitting still and screening out other needs and impulses. It is hard to imagine a five-year-old being willing or able to answer questions for three hours according to a strict idea of what the right answer will be, to understand that even though the task is tedious it is worth doing for some reward far down the road, and to resist the urge to transform the situation into something else altogether. Or, as another example, imagine an adult setting a table for dinner. The chances are good that the adult will begin and finish the task without lapsing into a small battle between two forks, as many four-year-olds might do. Children's behavior often shifts from one orientation to another. A child's talk interweaves imaginative with real-world pronouncements, and vacillates back and forth between more and less rational approaches to a situation or problem. Such interweaving and vacillation is one central way in which children's psychological experience is different from that of adults, and explains in part why it often appears messy or irrational.

UNEXPECTED MOMENTS FROM REAL CHILDREN

Though the child's inner life may often seem inaccessible to the researcher or casual observer, it peeks out now and then. Consider the following description. A five-year-old child, Sam, was standing in the kitchen, chatting with a member of his extended family and casually surveying the kitchen counter. Lying on the countertop was, among other vegetables, a cucumber with a somewhat rotten tip. Suddenly, as if out of nowhere, Sam uttered the following words: "My harmless inside heart turned green because I stabbed myself and it rotted because it could no longer live without being in me." His babysitter was so struck at the unexpectedness of what he said that she wrote it down. But an example like this, which has a particularly poetic quality, and is somewhat inscrutable, is hardly unique. Many young children between the ages of two and five use words to express unusual ways of thinking about experience. Kornei Chukovsky's classic book *From Two to Five* documents the pervasiveness and importance of young children's language play.[5] Sometimes the language has less ambiguity and meter than Sam's utterance, but nevertheless reveals the ways in which the young child's mind may be different from an adult's. Recently a young colleague mentioned that when she walked into her three-year-old daughter's bedroom, the little girl said, "Do you see that table? A voice you can't hear is telling me that is not a table." If we can put aside our adult urge to jump to an immediate conclusion—for example, that the child is disturbed and hears voices, or that it is a meaningless though appealing moment of "childishness"—such moments can tell us a lot about the child's construction of reality.

These kinds of utterances probably contain a logic, or meaning, even if that meaning is not easy to decipher or is not accessible to reflection by the child. Everyone who has spent time around children has seen or heard a child do something surprising. What kinds of understanding can those moments lead us to? Do we dismiss these moments as charming quirks, or simply evidence that this particular child is artistic or precocious? It is possible that some of the most useful data about children's thinking are lost because we do not take such phenomena seriously enough. What did Sam mean when he said those words? What did his words reveal about the way he thinks? And finally, what circumstances, internal and external, gave rise to that burst of thought and words?

To understand what such a verbal construction might tell us, we can begin by describing the immediate context in which it was elicited and made. Sam was not asked to write a poem. He was not even in a storytelling situation. Certainly he was not in school. He was in his own kitchen, rambling on about a range of matters with various people in his family (a brother, his babysitter, and so on). He was milling about quite relaxed, with no apparent goal (he wasn't doing schoolwork or a chore, nor was he engaged in any clear-cut play activity). He was using his body to explore the room by walking, jumping, and touching various objects. He was also using his body to express his thoughts and varying levels of interest and energy. That is, when excited by what the other person was saying, he listened with rapt attention. When talking to his babysitter about his day at kindergarten, he gesticulated and hopped on one foot. When he made his cucumber pronouncement, he had been idly leaning on the edge of the counter, doing nothing in particular, except looking and perhaps touching the vegetables lying there. The poem, if that is what it is, was created spontaneously, in the flow of other activities.

The spontaneity of Sam's production brings us to a second important point. His words merged a fairly prosaic and accurate (consensual) representation of everyday reality with a more fantastic and playful take on the situation. That is, within three phrases he managed to incorporate some image or association of a green cucumber, the rotting tip that he saw in front of him, and a fanciful and dramatic account of a person's heart. It is a classic example of a child using words to fulfill what British psychologist Michael Halliday called the ideational and communicative functions of language.[6] The words create and give life to an image, the ideational function, and at the same time quite dramatically communicate that thought to others, the communicative function. Thus, this example gives a feeling for the interconnectedness of the inner and outer worlds of childhood—thought and emotion, words and perception, reality and fantasy are all dynamically intertwined in the child's behavior and his experience. Sam's perception of the rotting cucumber, the images this gave rise to, and the freedom of words and movement afforded him by the situation all help explain how and why he said what he said.

But the example also illustrates the complexities, the seeming unruliness, of the child's inner thought. In trying to articulate how different disciplines attempt to understand autobiographical memory the literary critic Daniel Albright said, "Psychology is a garden, literature is a wilderness."[7] He meant, I believe, that psychology seeks to make patterns, find regularity, and ultimately impose order on human experience and behavior. Writers, by contrast, dive into the unruly, untamed depths of human experiences. What he said about understanding memory can be extended to our questions about young children's minds. If we psychologists are too bent on identifying the orderly pattern, the regularities of children's minds, we may miss an essential and pervasive characteristic of our topic: the child's more unruly and imaginative ways of talking and thinking. It is not only the developed writer or literary scholar who seems drawn toward a somewhat wild and idiosyncratic way of thinking; young children are as well. The psychologist interested in young children may have to venture a little more often into the wilderness in order to get a good picture of how children think. Once there, she will find that the idiosyncrasy and the flow back and forth between genres captured in Sam's cucumber narrative are the rule, not the exception.

Let me give another example, one that shows how quickly children can slide from one mode of experiencing to another. This example involves an eight-year-old boy and his father, who told me the story.

> We were sitting together in our living room. Actually I was lying on the floor, and he was sitting at my side, looking down at me. He was looking over the titles of our entire collection of Ian Fleming's James Bond books, a boxed set lying on the floor between his legs. He was deciding which he liked best, and for what reasons. He asked me which my favorite one was, and I answered, "*From Russia with Love.* Which is your favorite?" He responded, "*For Your Eyes Only.* I think I really like it best because of the song," at which point he broke out into the title song from the movie (Sheena Easton singing "For Your Eyes Only"). He sang with a great deal of drama and expression, gesticulating with his hands. Then suddenly, as he neared the end of the song phrase, his hand switched gestures, and started an abrupt, sharp poking action toward my eyes, while he said in an aggressive, sharp tone with a wild look in his own eyes, "Poke out your eyes, poke out your eyes." Just as abruptly, he dropped his hand, ended his tune/chant, smiled, and waited to pick up the quieter conversation about movies and books.

In the space of just a few minutes, this little boy had shifted from a fairly direct conversation with his father about some books, to imitating a pop singer, to playfully enacting some sort of violent impulse, and back again to the original quiet conversation. This anecdote illustrates how easily and quickly children slip in and out of various orientations and modes of behaving, and the context of this example reminds us that it happens in unexpected moments in everyday life.

These vivid instances, the kind any parent could recount if asked, stand out and are retold because they are thought of as cute, odd, or impressive. But what of the more everyday, prosaic behaviors of young children, seen in and out of research settings? Much of young children's everyday behavior falls under the research radar and is quickly forgotten as just small, everyday moments of children's actions and words. In order to improve the lens through which we see children, it is essential to identify the motivations driving any given piece of research, because these motivations influence the method used and, in turn, which aspects of the child will be considered salient, and which will be made invisible. Interestingly, the answer to the question "Why study children?" is not always as obvious or simple as one might think.

WHY STUDY CHILDREN?

Why should we want to know what a child thinks and feels, or how he experiences the world around him? We don't all study children for the same reasons. Moreover, the questions one asks are determined by the kind of answers one deems valuable. The motivations for studying children, and the kinds of questions asked, fall into several clusters—the most familiar of which date back to Jean Piaget.

Piaget, perhaps the most famous psychologist to study the development of young children, was the founder of a vast and influential group of investigators.[8] His original motivation is worth taking note of, because it shaped everything about the work he did, and the work generated by his theories. Piaget did not begin his career with an interest in children. Trained as a natural scientist, he did his early research and writing about mollusks. While still a young man, he became fascinated with the nature of scientific thought itself. How is it that human beings are able to categorize, develop taxonomies, and devise rules and principles from the messy experiences of everyday observations and encounters? This led him to an interest in how it is we developed such forms of thinking. Piaget studied children because he wanted to understand the underlying structure of scientific thought. Like many scientists, he believed that finding the origins of scientific thought, and watching the development of the process, would tell him about the nature of the process itself. Seeing that we don't start life capable of physics or algebra, he reasoned that if he watched as babies grew to children, and children to adults, he would "catch" the process of scientific thought as it unfolded. As developmental psychologist Joseph Glick has put it, he was interested in the mind "chez l'enfant" (housed in the infant). In other words, he was not particularly interested in children—their emotional lives, their education, or their potential to become better citizens.[9]

A perusal of current journals in child development will show that, by contrast, many contemporary psychologists are interested in ensuring that children will grow up into smart, good, psychologically stable, or altruistic people. The implicit long-term goal of many researchers is to ensure a good end state—a smart, kind, responsible, industrious, obedient adult. In other words, one school of psychologists cares about the origins of thinking, and another the origins of civilized behavior. The majority of educational research focuses little on the actual experiences of childhood, and almost completely on whatever outcome a given practice, or lack of intervention, might lead to. Beginning perhaps with studies carried out on the wild boy of Aveyron in the early 1800s, a great deal of research has been concerned with identifying the powerful shapers of development. When Jean Itard and others reported on what the wild boy could learn, and whether he would or could become more civilized once living with humans, their underlying interest was whether his earliest experiences without humans would shape him for life.[10]

There is a continuing preoccupation in the field of developmental psychology with the question of how malleable we are, what kinds of experiences are most likely to shape our adult behavior, and what aspects of our selves are impervious to influence during childhood. For example, are we born knowing how to think in numbers, talk, work together, and understand the feelings of another? Do we learn these things from our elders? Can we be changed through child-rearing practices or education? Many of the most pervasive questions fueling child development research concern environmental influences, genetic influences, and individual differences. All of this research in one way or another is directed at figuring out how and why we turn out the way we do as adults. In other words, these researchers are studying children to learn more about adults (and eventually how to get children to be competent and civilized adults). These motivations lead to certain kinds of empirical questions, which in turn guide researchers in what they see when they look at children. What they see affects us all.

OUR METHODS SHAPE THE CHILD WE SEE

In his classic book on cognitive processes, Ulric Neisser described the ways in which people develop "cognitive schema," plans and expectations that they build up from experiences in the world, which constrain and direct their subsequent perceptions of environments.[11] This is as true of researchers gathering data as it is of everyone else. The data we gather constrain and direct what we see when we look at children. For the most part, psychologists work with the premise that the data and conclusions derived from their experiments will help us understand children in everyday situations. The sequence usually goes something like this: a process, mechanism, or change is identified in a set of experiments. Further experiments are designed to allow the original researcher, or others in the field, to look even more closely at the particular mechanism or behavior. Their focus on a certain process or target behavior leads them to construct situations that will elicit those behaviors, and their coding systems focus them only on the behaviors that seem relevant to the process of interest. Eventually, researchers and consumers of research begin to feel that they can see the process or mechanism in everyday behaviors.

Developmental psychologist John Flavell, for example, has done considerable research fleshing out Piaget's argument that young children pay attention to appearances, and could easily be fooled about the real nature or identity of something. In a famous demonstration, Flavell used a confederate, a cat named Maynard, to test children's ability to see through an organism's superficial appearance to discover its "real" identity. Children would play with Maynard for a little while. Then they would encounter just the front part of Maynard, who now wore the mask of a vicious dog. Three-year-old children were scared, insisting that now Maynard was a mean dog. Six-year-olds scoffed and were certain it was still Maynard the cat, only wearing a mask that made him look like a dog, while four- and five-year-olds were confused.[12] This experiment gave heft to Piaget's original insights, and for many researchers and teachers alike, cemented the notion that young children cannot distinguish between appearance and reality. As a result, most well-trained early childhood educators will tell you that preschoolers should not have to participate in Halloween parades and so on because they will be freaked out by seeing people in masks. What Flavell demonstrated in a lab eventually affected the way nursery school teachers viewed their students.

Often, the way an experiment is set up confirms the findings of earlier work. But sometimes a change in the experimental approach allows researchers to reconsider old truths. For instance, several years ago psychologist Catherine Rice and her colleagues set up a slightly different kind of experiment to test children's distinctions between appearance and reality. She asked each three- to four-year-old child in the experiment to help her trick another adult by pretending that a sponge, which looked just like a rock, was really a rock. While preparing the trick, the experimenter asked each subject a series of questions about whether the object was really a rock, what the dupe (the other adult) would think when he came into the room and saw the item, and so forth. The children's comments made it clear that in this context they understood very well that though the item looked like a rock it was really a sponge, and they even understood why the other adult might be fooled. So, while children may not always distinguish between reality and appearance, Rice and her colleagues have shown that children can do so when they are in a situation that makes such a distinction meaningful to them.[13] Children's abilities, then, are not consistent. When children are interested in the problem, or the solution matters to them, they may seem (and be) smarter than when they find the problem uninteresting or irrelevant. The example of Rice's study shows that any given experiment may constrain or distort our picture of a child's abilities. An ingenious change in method can elicit a whole new kind of behavior, which in turn changes our view of children. Psychologists can take these examples simply as a caution to exert great care in designing laboratory experiments. I would argue, however, that the implications are larger. Taken together, a wide range of experiments demonstrating the powerful influence of context and the child's interpretation of the setting on the child's behavior suggests that perhaps our fundamental understanding of children needs to be rethought.

Sometimes the way a child functions in an experiment is surprising and leads to as many new questions as it does answers. When I was a graduate student, I had a professor who studied the development of children's mathematical knowledge. He had many graduate students collecting data with him on a range of well-thought-out, interconnected studies that showed how children come to identify shapes, see correspondences, and cluster their mathematical knowledge. Our favorite story about his research program, however, had to do with one particular incident. One of the graduate students had gone to a school to test some young subjects on a long list of items having to do with matching shapes and making judgments about size, contour, and other mathematical matters. The graduate student was doing his experiment in a small room in the school, taking each child for about forty-five minutes (it was a long battery of questions and tasks). One four-year-old boy was in the room with him, sorting the shapes and answering the questions. After about twenty minutes, and midway through the battery of tasks, the experimenter set out a new array of shapes to be sorted, and asked the little boy to solve the problem. The little boy looked at the array, looked up at the experimenter, got down on all fours, and started to growl at the experimenter. We used to laugh about that story. To us, it revealed the complete disjuncture between what researchers were interested in (the development of processes housed within the child's mind) and the real child. How could they think they were finding out about how children solve math problems with a task that made a child want to growl? A situation that makes you want to growl is eliciting and possibly shutting down thoughts that may or may not coincide with the cognitive processes adults identify as being central to the development of mathematical thinking. In other words, at the moment that a child, sitting in a room with a strange adult, looks down at a set of cards with colored geometric shapes on them, what is he thinking and feeling? What impulses are at the foreground, and what kinds of processes are at work? I would guess that this little boy was feeling bored, anxious, and frustrated. He wanted to move. He wanted to detach from the activity. He felt totally disengaged from the adult. He wanted to . . . growl like a lion. Not only was that one lost data entry for the study. It should have, and could have, reminded the experimenter that children do not think mathematically in a vacuum. They think mathematically while feeling, acting, and sensing. When Catherine Rice took into account what might make an appearance versus reality distinction interesting and meaningful to a child, she discovered that young children had an ability we had not identified before. When the little boy growled in the math study, perhaps the researchers should have tried to devise math tasks that engaged children in a way that tapped their mathematical interests more fully. The danger with not doing so is that the picture one builds of children is inaccurate.

It is not only that our data can constrain what we see, but that over time, our model of what children are becomes an artifact of the studies we have done. Let me give an example of research methods that directly shape the kind of model we construct. For many years researchers (and the general public) have been interested in gender differences. Psychologists have tried to answer two connected questions: What differences are there between little girls and boys, and how significant are these differences? The usual approach researchers take is to document some kind of behavior (ability at math, amount of time spent talking, vocabulary size, engagement in storytelling, rough-and-tumble play, and so on) and then look to see if girls perform differently than boys. For instance, do boys or girls tend to solve more math problems, or do boys solve a certain kind of math problem more quickly and easily than do girls? Do girls' stories about the past include information that boys' stories do not? Are boys, on the whole, more active than girls?

Some studies of this issue have brought boys and girls, one at a time, into a lab and asked them to solve a range of mathematical problems. The average boys' score has been found to be higher than the average girls' score on certain kinds of mathematically related skills (for instance, mentally rotating a figure or image). Or, to take another example, children have been invited, one at a time, to tell a story about something that has happened to them in the past. On average, girls are more likely to describe emotions than are boys.

The trouble is, as developmental psychologist Eleanor Maccoby has shown, this research often rests on the assumption that the difference resides in the individual. In order to question that assumption, Maccoby has taken a different approach. She has looked at groups of boys, groups of girls, and groups of boys and girls together. What she has found is that the differences between boys and girls are strengthened when they are in mixed-gender groups. For instance, girls tend to stay closer to the teacher when there are boys in the room. When they are in mixed-gender groups, children veer toward others of the same sex. When in those same-sex subgroups, their gender differences are exaggerated. This suggests that to understand the development of gender differences we have to think of the phenomenon as interpersonal rather than intrapersonal. The extent to which a girl manifests "girlish" behavior (such as staying close to the teacher, not dominating a discussion, taking up little physical space) will vary as a function of who else is in the room.[14] What is of special interest to me, however, is the way in which Maccoby's work shows that the method a researcher uses can have a strong effect on the conclusions and ultimately the theory that is offered. If you tend to measure children one by one, for example, you are likely to end up with a theory that focuses on differences between individuals. But when children are looked at in groups, as Maccoby did, it suddenly becomes clear that the theory itself has to take account of groups.

One of the most powerful tools of developmental psychology has been our ability to test children at different ages and compare the results between the two groups (say, three-year-olds and five-year-olds). In fact, this method has provided the great bulk of our information about development, by allowing us to pinpoint just what it is that changes, and when. For instance, we have learned in recent years that when a child is between the ages of four and five, something somewhat mysterious but certainly important shifts in their overall approach to thinking and solving mental problems. We have learned that this shift is apparent in a wide range of activities, no matter what the background or experience of the child, and is fairly impervious to training or other interventions. In other words, on all sorts of tasks four-year-olds almost always perform one way, and five-year-olds another. Five-year-olds seem almost magically to have gained certain kinds of cognitive skills that make them able to solve problems they couldn't just six months earlier. Our identification of critical moments in development, however, still leaves a big black hole with regard to how those changes occur, and under what conditions.

As one example of this, for years language researchers tended to focus on three stages of young children's language skills: prelinguistic, first words, and multiword phrases. Often researchers compared some aspect of the child's language by collecting data at two ages, for instance, twelve months and twenty-four months. A comparison of the language samples would typically show that some important leap had been made (for instance, the twelve-month-olds typically used one word at a time, while the twenty-four-month-olds used multi-word phrases with syntax). One group of psychologists argued, however, that the real developmental story lay between those stages. By drawing on the research of others, as well as by presenting new data, these psychologists showed that children were not magically jumping from single-word utterances to sentences. Instead, between twelve and twenty-four months children demonstrated what some researchers have called transitional phenomena. At some point between twelve and twenty-four months, children in this study would begin stringing single words together in a way that went beyond single words, but did not yet constitute grammatical multiword phrases. The child's intonation, and the relationships among the words, created some meaning beyond the individual meanings of the words, even though the children did not yet have command of syntax.[15] This way of conceptualizing early language development puts more emphasis on transition and less emphasis on discrete levels or stages of development. In looking at children's language between the major milestones, researchers found the steps by which children gradually shift from one kind of language skill to the next. The method of comparing performance between two age groups led to one conceptualization of development, and when a new method was introduced, a new model of development became possible. It is important to note, however, that in this example, as with the Maccoby example, the new method was more naturalistic, and messier, than the older method.

My point here is not to discuss the development of gender differences or word forms but to give two examples of how the methods one uses to look at children (or anything for that matter) have a strong influence on what one can discover, and ultimately on the kind of theory that the data support. Often what is "cleanest" or easiest to look at empirically does not necessarily answer the questions we really care about. About once a year someone (usually a psychologist) mentions to me the story of the drunkard who is looking for his watch under the lamppost, not because that is where he actually dropped his watch, but because the light is better there. What I find funniest about this joke is that even though we all know that story, we continue to look under the lamppost. The easiest way to measure children's thinking may not lead us to the fullest and most powerful understanding of how they think and experience the world.

Not all researchers see children as future adults. There are some who consider the child and the child's mind to be topics of intrinsic importance without looking past to some other endpoint. What does the child feel and think? How does the world look to a three-year-old? These students of human experience and behavior may or may not have other motives (helping children learn, understanding the origins of symbolic functioning), but they do in fact look at the whole child in real settings. Dennie Wolf is a good example of this kind of researcher. While her overarching interest is the processes by which we become complex symbol users, her research focuses on the ways in which young children experience the world of symbols and symbol making.[16] Not surprisingly, psychologists such as Wolf tend to look at children in real-life settings, and often offer detailed descriptions as part of their data. For instance, Wolf has offered careful descriptions of the different styles of play that children employ. She has found that given a range of toys, and the chance to initiate play on their own (in nursery schools and at home), some children can be described as "patterners" who are more interested in the shape of toys and what they can make with the toys, and some are "dramatists" who are more interested in using toys to enact scenarios. Such close descriptions, across various settings and over time, describe what real children do and how they differ from one another; they also offer insights into what various activities mean to the children themselves.

We can learn something about this approach from psychologists who study children's behavior across cultures. Suzanne Gaskins and her colleagues have been watching the play of children in a small community in Mexico for over twenty-five years. She has found that their play is quite different from the play of white middle-class children in the United States, though she has also found some interesting similarities.[17] For instance, there seems to be much less imaginative scene enactment in the Mexican community, though children in both cultures engage in role-playing in familiar domestic settings (by playing house, for instance). Gaskin, who has been careful not to form too many hypotheses, and who is ready to sit on the sidelines and watch for long periods of time over an even longer span of study, has offered an extremely useful understanding of how another community of children might play, and what this play might mean to them. Through such research, we can begin to learn not only what children really do when they play, but also how this play varies from individual to individual as well as between communities and cultures.

If one wants to understand young children (rather than a process housed in young children), one is likely to need full and detailed accounts of young children in action. But as the two earlier examples suggest, children are always acting and experiencing within a specific context. While researcher Barbara Rogoff has shown how adults shape and define children's activities, there is another equally important piece of context that requires consideration: How the child interprets the situation is as much a part of the context as the place, the people, and the activities themselves.[18] This is as true of the laboratory context as it is of the playground or the living room.

HOW CHILDREN INTERPRET SITUATIONS

While we are busy interpreting children's behavior in various experimental settings, the children are busy interpreting the experiment, or at least construing the situation in ways that differ from our construals. The feelings, thoughts, and concerns that influence a child in a given situation may have a strong effect on what they do or say, and hence what we make of their abilities. When my eldest son Jake was four, we went for his annual check-up at our local pediatrician. Jake had recently undergone ear surgery, and so he had a more ominous feeling about doctors' offices than another child might have had. We were asked to fill out a developmental inventory as part of the check-up. In one section I was supposed to ask Jake to draw a person on the sheet. Then I was supposed to look and see how many arms and legs his figure had, as one indication of his level of cognitive development. Jake's figure had no arms and legs. He drew a nice round body, cute little head with eyes and a mouth, but no limbs. I like to think that under other circumstances I would have been interested in and admiring of his unique rendition of a person. But since he was being evaluated and since my degree in developmental psychology is irrelevant when it comes to my own children, I was dismayed to see that he fell very short on the developmental schedule. I said nothing to him about the picture, but continued on with the other tasks and questions on the sheet. As we stood up to go into the doctor's room, filled-out sheet in hand, Jake said somewhat offhandedly, "See that man I drew? He used to have two legs and two arms, but the doctor cut them off!" According to the inventory, Jake would have been assessed at one developmental level, and then, if the evaluator had heard the thoughts that went with his actions, a different level a moment later. But more generally, this example reminds us that there are few acts, even for a four-year-old, that aren't caused, shaped, or accompanied by the child's own range of ideas, interpretations, and images.

One of the most important uncharted aspects of the child's mind concerns the ways in which the young child interprets the situations and tasks she encounters, in laboratories and in everyday life. What a child thinks the meaning of a task is will have a huge effect on how she functions, and thus on our assessment of that child (or age group's) abilities. In one of the first and best demonstrations of this phenomenon, the British psychologists Martin Hughes and Margaret Donaldson showed that children do not always interpret Piagetian tasks the way that Piaget and his followers supposed. For instance, in the famous three mountain tasks, the five-year-old is seated on one side of a three-dimensional model of mountains with small scenes and characters placed on it. A doll is placed on the opposite side of the model. The experimenter asks the child to tell him what the doll sees. The young children whom Piaget and his followers questioned were unable to describe the scene from the doll's point of view; instead they described only what they themselves saw. This was evidence, Piagetians claimed, for the child's cognitive egocentrism. The child implicitly assumes that everyone sees things from her perspective. When Hughes and Donaldson made a few small but important modifications to the nature of the task, however, the results were very different. The researchers explained to each young subject that a small child had stolen some cookies, and that the "bobbies" were looking for the young thief. The child was then shown an area dissected by two screens, so that there were four chambers. Two toy policemen were placed at two adjacent walls. The researchers then asked each subject where the child would have to hide so as not to be seen by either police officer. Almost all five-year-old children could correctly solve this problem. This study showed that five-year-olds could take the perspective of another, given a situation that makes sense to them dramatically and thus visually.[19] In other words, children's understanding of the meaning and motives of a situation dramatically influences both the cognitive processes they use and the skills they can demonstrate within a given situation. The simple message from this example is that context matters a lot to young children. Since Hughes and Donaldson's elegant demonstration, literally thousands of studies have shown that Piaget's tasks shaped his conclusions, and that changing the task can often make a child look more competent at an earlier age than Piaget led us first to believe.

Another compelling example is an elegant study conducted by the Soviet psychologist Z. M. Istomina in the mid-twentieth century. Istomina was not satisfied with the data showing that five-year-olds had only a small memory capacity for lists of items, and little or no ability to deliberately remember things (if one reads a list of words to a five-year-old, he or she is likely to remember only a few items on the list, compared to the performance of a nine-year-old, who is likely not only to remember many more items on the list, but also to use all kinds of strategies such as rehearsal, grouping like items together, and so on). She guessed that five-year-olds might remember more if they had a good reason for remembering. So she set up a play store in the childhood center where she did her research. Children had to make up a grocery list in one room, and then go to the other room to "shop" for the items. Lo and behold, five-year-olds remembered far more items, and used more deliberate strategies for remembering, when they were playing store than when they were simply subjects in a list recall experiment.[20]

The case has been made that such studies show we need more ingenious research methods. In fact a great deal of energy has gone into devising tasks that allow a child to "look as smart as he really is." Hence we see experiments in which even a baby can add, by responding differently to pictures of objects that "add" the number of objects the baby has previously seen. But I think there is a more important point to be learned from such research, which is that at the most basic level children always respond to the situation at hand. The context of a task has a lot to do with how children interpret the task, how much effort they put into it, and consequently what cognitive processes or skills they are able to access in order to solve the task. It is not simply that we will see how smart children are if we give them tasks they find relevant; more importantly, their cognitive skills vary as a function of dynamics such as interest, relevance, and the presence of others. Such variation, and responsiveness to context, is not a wrinkle on our picture of children's development, but must be seen as an essential and important characteristic of the young child.

WHEN CHILDREN ARE OPAQUE

What children say can reveal to us what they think and how they experience an experimental setting, or even how they experience the world. But often their words and actions are not very transparent. Instead we need to probe, analyze, and decipher in order to harvest the information embedded in their behavior. Often any given piece of behavior is complex and reflects a complex layering of feelings and thoughts.

By the time a child is four or five, a good part of her thinking is oblique or covert. That is, often children, like adults, find ways of burying the meaning of their statements, stories, and communications so that it is not obvious for the listener or reader. Take, for instance, the young child who watches her mother care for a dying friend. She says nothing about what is going on, though she protests the frequent trips the mother makes to the city, two hours from home, where the sick friend lives. This is a young girl who read reluctantly at first, without ease. She was at the end of her eighth year before she could read a whole book. Yet during this seemingly nonliterate period of her development, she wrote the following poem:

THE OCEAN
the ocean.
I can see you in the ocean.
Even if you're gone.
Even if you live with the angels.
I can still see you in the ocean.
I can still see your beautiful eyes in
the ocean. I can still see the olive
green in your skin. Because I always knew
that was your color

This little girl clearly has turbulent and subtle thoughts about her mother's friend. The mother had said that when she looks at the ocean she feels the presence of her dead friend. So when the little girl writes this poem, she invokes her mother and expresses her need to internalize her mother. She is thus also showing her anxiety about her separations from her mother. One salient feature of her mother's relationship with the friend is that her mother is white and her friend was black. This means that the prominence of color and skin color in the poem also reflects the child's rumination on her mother and her mother's friendship. A cognitive psychologist would, no doubt, object to the highly interpretive clinical nature of the foregoing comment. But without understanding the meanings of this poem, one cannot really appreciate its cognitive features. To dismiss it because a poem falls outside the realm of empirical psychology is to miss valuable data about what is essential to human beings—the making of meaning. The challenge is to find a way to understand these layers of a child's experience, rather than to find good ways of circumventing them. To understand those layers, one must be ready to deal with the highly intertwined nature of children's experience.

Some researchers have adopted approaches to their research that allows for just that kind of multilayered understanding. Developmental psychologist Alyssa McCabe has described her research on narrative development as a "literary analysis of children's stories."[21] This implies that children's narratives, speech, and play require textual consideration, and that such work can lead us deeper into the inner life of the child. But just as language and play converge and diverge rapidly in a few moments of a child's behavior, so too do the child's thoughts and feelings suffuse one another. This interaction is equally important for us to understand more fully.

THE INTERPLAY OF THOUGHT AND FEELING

Some interesting studies have shown that in fact emotional and cognitive processes drive one another during the early years, often in rather straightforward ways. Peggy Miller has shown that children are more likely to tell stories to their parents about accidents and other sympathy-arousing experiences than about more mundane or anger-arousing experiences.[22] The desire for sympathetic response drives the narrative process. Robyn Fivush and Judith Hudson have both shown that three-year-olds recall emotionally packed experiences differently than more prosaic or emotionally bland events.[23] Paul Harris argues that involvement in a fictional world can arouse strong feelings. In one study he told a story to children involving a protagonist much like the child (same gender, age, and so on). Some of the children were encouraged to feel what the main character felt, while others were encouraged to remain detached. A third group was simply told to listen carefully. The story involves a sad event in which a family moves away from a city, leaving close friends behind. Whereas all the children reported feeling cheerful before the story began, those children who had been encouraged to immerse themselves in the fictive world were the most likely to report feelings of sadness afterward. In addition, when recalling the story they were more likely to use terms conveying sadness, even though their overall recall of the story was comparable to the other two groups.[24] Harris uses this and similar studies to argue that while young children can and do distinguish between reality and fantasy, once they enter a "fictive world" their real feelings can be aroused. We will return later to the discussion of the distinctions children make between fantasy and reality. For now, it is interesting to see that researchers have shown that children's cognitive processes (their ability, for instance, to remember or to reason about something) and their feelings are connected in ways that go beyond the obvious. The point here is not merely that a very upset child may not be rational. The way a child solves a problem, recalls the past, and organizes boundaries around his experience is part and parcel of the emotions he is feeling at any given time. Examples from the work of psychologists like Harris and Fivush remind us that there is rarely a cognitive problem that does not elicit feeling in the problem solver. But that insight should be the beginning of our investigations, not simply a conclusion to be set aside. Doing so could be compared to a medical researcher, having understood that chronic back pain is intricately tied to the mental state of the patient, proceeding to construct experiments in which the patient's mental state is considered "noise," "irrelevant," or in some way a variable to be held constant.

The work of people such as Harris and Fivush not only suggests that we need to learn more about how feelings and thoughts shape one another, but tells us that the connection must be taken into account whenever we design studies, or draw conclusions about children's behavior.

In the earlier example of the girl who wrote the poem about her mother's friend, the girl's advanced literary skill (use of imagery, phrasing, words, and sounds to convey a potent meaning) was triggered by strong feelings and a vivid experience. A child who still barely reads suddenly writes with great ease because she has something important to say, and in saying it, she does something important (connects to her mother).

But this example also shows that the girl's concerns, as well as her skills for symbolizing these concerns, are not manifested in any direct way in her actions, conversations, or schoolwork. The opaqueness of children's feelings and abilities is important to acknowledge as we think about how to investigate the child's mind. Take for example the opening quote to Roger Brown's landmark book, *A First Language*. It is from one of their three subjects, Eve, before she was three: "I hafta pee-pee just to pass the time away."[25] The child's quite concrete and practical thoughts about pee-peeing, a major focus of the toddler's life, are interwoven with something more idiosyncratic and lyrical. As Kornei Chukovksy argues in his underappreciated book *From Two to Five*, young children are astonishingly inventive in their use of language.[26] And it is probably the rule rather than the exception for this lyricism and invention to be at its most evident when the child is talking about important matters, even when those matters seem prosaic, rational, or goal oriented (such as the need for a toddler to pee).

Young children not only intertwine the lyrical with the rational or prosaic. Their attempts to offer socially appropriate and circumscribed responses often blend with their more impulsive, fantasy-driven responses as well. Their responses (verbal or behavioral) are layered and complex and cannot be separated from the impulses that help inspire them.

Recently I was told about a young boy (perhaps six or seven) who was acting in a dramatic film about three years ago. I have seen the film, and the boy's acting is a marvel—winsome, spontaneous, and totally convincing. While making the film, however, the director had a great deal of difficulty because every time the little boy said his lines, he fondled his penis. When the director asked the young actor to keep his hand away from his penis, the little boy could no longer say his lines. The director's wise solution was to film the child only from the waist up. Again, a fairly rational, deliberate, task-oriented process (saying lines in a movie) is totally infused, for this young boy, with other sensations and impulses. Claudia Lewis gives a wonderful example of this in her paper "Our Native Use of Words." She describes an early childhood classroom in which one boy is asked to tell the group what sound a dinosaur makes. In order to give that information he seems compelled to stand up from the seated circle, stretch his arms up, and shriek "Yeeeee!" The teacher thanks him and then asks if all the children can sing the song "Old Macdonald Had a Farm" (and on his farm they had a dinosaur), sitting down. Yet when they get to that verse the boy jumps up once again, stretching as high as possible and shrieking "Yeeeee!" Lewis writes, "Piaget has said that to silence the child's tongue is to silence his thinking. We might add: to immobilize his body is to silence his language and thought."[27] How can we begin to understand the steps the mind takes to solve a given problem, if we think those steps unfold separately from the feelings, images, and impulses with which they are intertwined?

BENEFITS OF A NATURALIST APPROACH

Too often we harbor the misconception that a child has one pure or absolute level of ability or knowledge, just waiting to be elicited. But it is often much more valuable to find out what a child does rather than simply what she can do under certain circumstances. Here we turn to a long but undernourished tradition in developmental psychology.

Oddly enough, developmental psychologists have given short shrift to an invaluable step in trying to understand young children: careful detailed descriptions of children playing, eating, and working at home, in day care centers, and in other communal spaces. The field began with such descriptions and contains pockets of such accounts such as James Sully's *Studies of Childhood,* written in the early part of the twentieth century, and diary studies such as those conducted by Charles Darwin, Jean Piaget, and Michael Halliday.[28] But aside from these periodic accounts, there are remarkably few careful and full records of children in real situations, functioning in real time. This approach, often referred to as ecological or naturalistic, is fairly unusual and often not taken seriously by developmental psychologists. When one compares the field of child development to other sciences that study animals, one finds a relative paucity of naturalists—observers who set out to meticulously document their subject (cranes, icebergs, wolves, or in this case, children) in its natural setting. It is more respectable to study primates in their natural habitats than human children in their homes.

As developmental psychologist Susan Sugarman has argued, at some point during the past one hundred years, the value of describing child development got left behind. As she puts it, though Piaget started with a lot of minute and illuminating descriptions of his own children, too quickly he let his ideas about development (his theory) guide and limit his observations. "Insofar as the most basic agenda of the discipline is to describe the child's mind and how it changes, then there are significant ways in which neither Piaget nor many of his successors have carried out this agenda. Piaget aimed to carry it out, but instead imposed an adult grid on the children's behavior, and introduced other arbitrary assumptions about how they think."[29] The importance of creating a full and detailed description of children was lost as a goal of child researchers. As a result, our descriptions are limited, as are the conclusions they might lead us to about the nature of and constraints on children's thinking. Sugarman's point is that if you always set a child up to do a task in which you have already decided what the underlying processes are, you are doomed to miss what might be really going on. Thus she, and a handful of others, such as Barbara Rogoff, have done studies of what she calls everyday cognition, and have constructed detailed accounts of children as they solve everyday problems. For instance, the way children count money when they are actually selling something often is different than the way they count when they are asked to do so in an experiment, when an adult is constructing and interpreting the child's activities. The social meaning of a child's play and work must be taken into account.

The following story illustrates the ways in which more naturalistic and careful collections (for instance of drawings, utterances, or play sequences) and descriptions of children may have a lot to tell us about children. Recently I was on a long train ride. Just behind me sat a couple with their three-year-old daughter. She talked for almost the entire two-hour ride, asking an unending stream of questions: "What's the train doing NOW? When are we gonna be in New York CITY . . . Chug chig a choo choo. Chug a chug a poo poo. How COME we have ta switch trains. How COME we have to switch trains. Will this train cry when we leave it? Why WON'T this train be sad? How come we are getting up NOW?" and so on. The parents were quiet, only answering every fourth question or so, and then only briefly. Clearly they were used to such a barrage of questions. But I, listening, was struck by the potential wealth of information her monologue offered an interested psychologist. As I sat there watching her parents barely notice her torrent of questions (I would have probably done the same if it had been my child), I wondered which of our theories of childhood would best explain her behavior. The answer is that there is not much in the most current and popular research on young children that deals with such behavior. The best effort, and the best example, is in the book *The Scientist in the Crib.*[30]

Written by three developmental psychologists, the book does an impressive job of summarizing, for researcher and lay reader alike, our most up-to-date understanding of how babies and toddlers try to understand the world's rules (particularly concerning inanimate objects). But just as the title suggests, it focuses very much on a rational world, understood in rational terms. The authors imagine the baby as a budding scientist making sense of an orderly world. The book does not try to account for the ways in which most young children blend an interest in the rules of the physical world with an interest in their own less constrained imaginative worlds, for instance, or the way in which their feelings about people and events dominate their understanding of those people and events.

I think the mismatch between current theories and the behavior of actual children also points to what remains unknown and misunderstood about young children's inner lives. We see a child just learning how powerful a tool language is, both pragmatically (to get attention and to engage other people) and cognitively (to understand things about the world that mystify her). Talking clearly feels good to her. She seems deeply absorbed by the act of constructing sentences—interested equally in their sounds as well as their meanings. Her "whys" and "whats" are like picks or wedges she uses to get herself deeper into the world of shared knowledge. As psychologist Michael Maratsos pointed out so long ago, it may seem amazing that a child this young has so much facility with language, but it is equally astonishing to see just how diligently and persistently she practices variations on a form—in this case the question form (how COME, WHY we don't have to, why DON'T we have to), and so forth.[31] In this little snippet of behavior we see a child trying to understand a range of phenomena—how a train ride works, what matters and what doesn't, how to get her parents to talk to her, how to structure why questions, and how to draw the line between things that feel and things that don't. All of this packed into a relatively "unimportant" two-hour stretch of her young life. It shows a child actively working on making sense of her social and physical environment. But it also shows a child who uses all strategies at her disposal—private and social, real world and fantasy, rational and playful.

The example above also shows a three-year-old employing several modes of functioning at once, or in quick succession. A researcher looking strictly at logical thinking would only find a third of this little girl's utterances useful. Another researcher focusing on play, imaginative thought, or make-believe might make use of a totally different third of the utterances. Furthermore, looking at utterances alone would leave out the portion of time that the child's body was heavily involved in her activity. Thus this seemingly banal stretch in a child's everyday life suggests that at least some of what is most important and interesting about a young child's mind appears too messy to understand using most conventional research tools. One would not see this litany of questions, language games, and commentary during a lab session employing one of the methods used these days. That is, asking a child to answer questions about a scenario involving puppets, hidden objects, or previously witnessed actions with a toy, or asking a child to explain why he answered a number of questions the way he did, might tell you a lot about the limits of that age group's ability to comment on their own intellectual processes, but would not reveal the kind of stream of questions children have about their daily experience, nor would it show you the multiplicity of purposes to which they put language in a given slice of time. In fact, looking at any one strand of this monologue would leave out what may be most interesting and revealing about it—the multilayered complexity of the child's mental processes. The account also suggests, I think, that all too often what is missed is an understanding of the rich and complex inner life of the child—not simply what they can do under some given conditions, but how they feel, what they think, and what they are inclined to do under the noisy conditions of real experience.

Two important features of a child's experience stand out both because they seem so important, and because too often research neglects them: time and place. Children function in time, and over time, and in almost every example I can think of, in or out of a lab, understanding what the child was thinking, or doing, involved seeing them over time. So for instance the child who growled at the researcher only did so after he had been in the lab room for over thirty minutes. Children who are solving math problems come up with new strategies when they spend enough time doing them, and in fact they take even more time to become aware of the strategies they are using. In everyday life as well, time ends up being central to the meaning of the phenomena. To understand what might be going on in the mind of the little girl on the train, one would have to have heard her ask all of those questions as they unfolded over the entire two hours.

By contrast, when the little boy uttered his poem about the cucumber it just popped out in a moment, though it was a fleeting moment, and might not have been produced had anything about the situation been different. If you hadn't been there, you would have missed it.

The second feature that must be taken seriously has to do with context. Nowadays context has become such a popular term that it is overly burdened with meaning. I mean a fairly modest or narrow interpretation of context: that watching a child alone will give you a very different impression than watching the child in a group of children all of the same age, and that this will look different than that same child in a mixed-age group. Why does this matter? Because we are situational creatures, responsive to the people who are in the room with us, and what kind of room it is. But during early childhood, when characteristics and ways of operating are in such flux, the role of others is even more important. So, for instance, a two-year-old in a room of two-year-olds will tell a very different developmental story than a two-year-old in a room with an experimenter, or alone with a set of toys.

Most scientists will argue at this point that it is our job to isolate one characteristic, trait, or process and examine it separately from other influences. For most of its existence the field of psychology has modeled itself on a certain kind of natural science, sometimes unpleasantly referred to as "hard science." This formal approach is based on the important principle that a great deal of certainty and specificity depends on controlling variables. If you want to know which kind of fertilizer works best on potatoes, the best experiment is one in which everything else is exactly the same (climate, earth, planting technique) and the only difference between plots of potatoes is the fertilizer. By the same token, if you want to study a child's ability to reason numerically, you might want to set up a situation in which all children are faced with a numerical situation or problem, and try your best to clear out any interference caused by individual variations in children's playfulness, strong feelings, personal interactions, and so on. This approach continues to yield important truths about young children. Without such carefully crafted and executed studies, for instance, we would not have learned that in fact babies as young as nine months are able to reenact a small set of actions that they have previously witnessed, suggesting that the building blocks of episodic memory appear earlier than we used to believe. Similarly, we would not know that infants as young as six months respond differently when they see a group of objects that matches the number of objects they have previously observed, suggesting that they have some rudimentary sense of quantity years before they can actually add. We would also not know that children are more likely to engage in aggressive behaviors right after they have participated in certain kinds of video games, regardless of their background or upbringing. What we have learned from such studies is considerable. The problem with focusing primarily on such methods, however, is that this approach may have also slowly and insidiously led us astray in the overall model we have of young children's minds. It is unlikely that most children ever approach a numerical problem in an emotional and imaginative vacuum. It may be that because we are scientists, we tend to assume that that's what children are trying to be too, able to think about a certain problem and put everything else (personal lives, immediate visceral reactions, and fantasies) aside. In trying to isolate their more scientific or rational thinking from other aspects of their experience, we may get a distorted view of the phenomenon. Recently a colleague told me, "It does continue to amaze me that most developmental psychologists know so little about children, even when they have some at home. I showed yesterday's class the film *Piaget on Piaget* and noted once again that the demonstration of the conservation of volume problem is off the wall. Any normal child of four would be more concerned, even worried about, the little blocks falling over than about whether his tower has the same quantity or volume as the model tower."[32] This is just one example of the way in which our questions constrain our findings.

The goal of more descriptive, naturalistic research is not simply to test the relative influence of a given variable on a specific outcome or behavior, but more importantly to develop well-articulated descriptions of the processes children use when encountering the world. Such descriptions can then be used to theorize about how the child thinks in a given situation, or when confronted with a given problem. Susan Sugarman's early research offers a good example of how important detailed descriptions can be in testing theories. Her early work was prompted by Piaget's claim that children between the ages of eighteen months and three years did not organize objects in the world into categories (categories that will later form the basis of concepts). She had the feeling that children might have more of a sense of grouping, or categories, than their final performance on a task might indicate. She set a whole bunch of blocks, which varied in shape and color, on a surface in front of a young toddler. Then she filmed the toddler's behavior as he or she surveyed them. What she found from repeating this experiment with many toddlers is that even if the toddlers weren't able, in the end, to group the blocks by color or shape, their hands moved over them in patterns that suggested they were being guided by principles of color and shape categories. The toddler's hand might touch a red block, then hover over another red block, then feel a third red block, before drifting over to a few of the blue blocks. In this case, watching and describing the toddlers' actions indicated to the researcher something that the result of a test might not tell her. Sugarman's aim was to show that children were using concepts to guide their movements before they were able to use those concepts to solve tasks. Their process as it unfolded in real time showed something different than any score on their final groups would reveal. Her work shows that close observations of young children have as much to offer us as beautifully designed experimental tasks—and that often a child will reveal what and how she is thinking through a sequence of behaviors. That is, we can learn a lot about the phenomenology of childhood from watching children in real settings.[33]

In presenting various scientific methods for studying children's behaviors, and by juxtaposing the results of these studies with behaviors of children in more everyday settings, I have argued that children may not be as rational and task-oriented as research has unwittingly led us to believe. Children interpret experimental settings, and those interpretations play a crucial role in shaping their behavior. Thus children's performance on a wide range of dimensions shifts when the context shifts (in experiments as well as in everyday life). And our view of children changes as a function of what we measure (the dependent variable).

A more naturalistically based account of children, one that takes their complex inner lives into account and may offer insights into the mind of this more changeable child, need not begin in a vacuum. One cannot begin to revise our approach to understanding children, or the view we have of children, without taking into account what has been learned already. In order to develop a detailed and multidimensional understanding of young children's minds, we need to take stock of what we already think and know about children, by drawing on nearly one hundred years of research and observation.

2 A Glance Backward

What Have We Learned about Children?

Too often we miss seeing, or taking seriously, behavior that holds rich clues to the child's mind. Sometimes our preexisting ideas about children function like blinders, preventing us from attending to the important data. It is equally true, however, that our ideas or theories about children help us see through the surface of their behavior to a deeper level. A theory works something like an X-ray machine, helping us to see the underpinning or armature of a child's actions and words. Each time I am intrigued by something a small child does or says, I ask myself what I know that can help me understand what I am observing. Invariably, in the face of real live childishness, I wonder what seven decades of research have taught us, and whether we have added to what we know, or changed what we know altogether. What have researchers, educators, and parents thought about the mind of the child over the past seventy years or so? Has our thinking changed in any important ways, and have new findings dramatically altered our models of the child's mind?

One could write vast books summarizing and detailing the many, increasingly focused, strands of research in developmental psychology. But rather than catalogue the huge and impressive array of research, in this chapter I will highlight some of the most important leaps and changes that have brought us to our current views. Much of that research and the views it has led to are captured by two contrasting metaphors. These metaphors do not neatly or completely encompass all the subtleties of seventy years of complex work. Instead they offer a heuristic for understanding a vast body of work, and help explain some of the unhelpful dichotomies we have inherited, and against which I argue later in the book. I will also describe what I consider to be the touchstone of psychological research on young children—the ideas and legacy of Piaget. Though many of his specific findings and claims have since been refuted, most research on children's minds is, in one way or another, a conversation with Piaget. The effect Piaget has had on subsequent developmental psychologists is similar to that described by literary critic Harold Bloom, in his classic book *The Anxiety of Influence*.[1] In describing the power previous great poets have had on those that followed, Bloom argued that giants within a field dominate the thoughts and concerns of those who come after them. Psychologists may not suffer the anxiety of poets, but certainly they bear the influence of the powerful scholars who preceded them.

THE WILD CHILD

Historically, there has been a strong tension between viewing young children as beasts, faeries, wild things, or criminals, and seeing them as small adults, machines, computers, or young scientists. Our knowledge about young children has developed along these two pathways, often as if the two bodies of knowledge, stemming from the two sets of metaphors, had little to do with one another.

There are two roots to the wild child metaphor. The first is the idea, captured in Jean-Jacques Rousseau's *Emile* (though also implied in Aristotle's epistemology) that the baby is born free and unfettered by any of the evils or abilities of the older child or adult.[2] The baby cannot read or think about philosophy, and is oblivious to social convention or responsibility. Rousseau gave us the image of the young child frolicking gaily and unself-consciously through the meadow, playing and pursuing his whims. A second, less theoretical and less bucolic conceptualization of children as wild came from Jean-Marc Itard's description of the Wild Boy of Aveyron, a key account for anyone interested in the history of developmental psychology.[3] In 1800 he took in a boy who appeared to have survived in the near wilderness with almost no human interaction. Itard saw it as a wonderful opportunity to find out just what the role of environment is in the development of the child. For example, how was it that the child could walk and manipulate objects, but not talk or manage everyday encounters with people? What could the child do and what could he be taught to do? Though Itard didn't subscribe to Rousseau's views (he was a follower of Locke), his story added another dimension to the view that childhood is best understood as a time of unadulterated wildness that becomes constrained, molded, or tamed by society.

The notion that we might actually get to see what a child is like who hasn't been molded by civilization continues to capture our lurid and puerile imaginations. Luckily these natural experiments are few and far between. Further, it will be no surprise to the reader to hear that in fact these natural experiments are mortally flawed because it is impossible to disentangle and thus evaluate the conditions that led to the baby's neglect and isolation, the emotional influence of such an impoverished and distorted environment, and the lack of specific kinds of input that we might want to investigate (language, cognitive skills, and so on). Years ago, there was great excitement as well as dismay among a group of psychologists when a little girl named Genie was discovered to have lived most of her life in isolated captivity in a room in her parents' home. The story, chronicled by Russ Rymer, is as illuminating about psychological research as it is about the horrible and fascinating experiences of this devastated little girl.[4] It was finally concluded that there was no way to tell whether Genie continued to seem so damaged (developmentally delayed, and seriously impaired) because she had been that way in the first place (some thought her father had imprisoned her because she seemed retarded as an infant) or whether her experiences of abuse and neglect had kept her from the input essential for development. Moreover, psychologists were almost totally unable to tease apart the emotional effects of abuse and neglect from the cognitive influences of such environmental impoverishment. In other words, even when such natural experiments present themselves, they have proven to yield muddy results at best. But as limited as the conclusions about Genie were, she offered psychologists a grim peek at an uncivilized (and uncivilizing) childhood, and fed a collective image of children as inherently wild creatures.

The idea persists that if we could only get a good approximation of the pure, unadulterated child, we could separate and measure the relative influences of environment and biology. The thinking and research that circles around this notion rests on the assumption that there is in fact a natural child who subsequently gets molded by his environment.

These notions of an impulse-driven child unhampered by conventions, but also unhampered by adultlike thought processes and knowledge, can be seen throughout the literature on child development. Though stories such as Itard's and Genie's are not of a piece (for instance, not all of the scientists who studied Genie would knowingly ascribe to a wild child theory of development), they have directly and indirectly contributed to, and are emblematic of, the assumption that children begin life in a natural state that is reshaped, with great effort, by society. The wild child metaphor has influenced the very behaviors and processes that psychologists have deemed important and consequently investigated. It has also shaped our views of children along several important dimensions. Three enduring lines of research that have in turn molded popular views of young children all can be traced, to some extent, to the wild child metaphor: the young child's tendency to seek what she wants at all costs, her need for attachment in early life, and her playfulness.[5]

Ruled by Impulse

Psychologists, parents, and teachers often view children as impulsive and pleasure seeking, unfettered by moral considerations and inhibitions. Rousseau's archetypal child comes across as freely gamboling through the fields, not yet deformed by the demands and corruptions of education and society. Although his view was put forth long ago, in the mid-1700s, some version of this image persists, though its interpretations and uses have gone through some sea changes. For instance, Rousseau's free child was open, happy, and curious, but also innocent of darker impulses associated with adulthood. In contrast, some views have suggested that the child is not simply free of adult worries and conventions, but also free of the adult's moral constraints and subterfuge—that is, the young child expresses passions that over time he learns to conceal. In 1997 the photographer Sally Mann published a book of photographs of young children (mostly her own children) that demonstrate this view. The children are seen standing, playing, or lolling around, naked or half-dressed. Each child is invariably lying on a porch, or leaning against a mossy tree, suggesting a world of almost animal-like existence, free from the watchful eyes of adult society.[6] The images are full of latent sexuality, and are disturbing at least to the modern eye. Her pictures, which were posed, generated a great deal of controversy when they were first published. Some felt that she was imposing sexuality onto the children. But the debate about her photographs revealed conflicting views of what children are really like. Like Louis Malle's film *Pretty Baby,* or Vladimir Nabokov's *Lolita,* Mann's photographs capture the idea that young children have a wild side.[7] In the style of Rousseau's Emile, Mann's children are surrounded by nature, free of adult constraints. But whereas Emile is light and innocent, uncorrupted by adulthood, Mann envisions children who contain and express some of the turbulent and wild feelings of adults. In novels such as William Golding's *Lord of the Flies* or Richard Hughes's *A High Wind in Jamaica,* the children act on violent impulses when they are given any kind of freedom from adult supervision.[8] Clearly neither Malle, Golding, nor Mann can prove that the children they depict have the turbulent or wild feelings suggested by the artists. But their work expresses an implicit idea about children that is shared by many, and that is supported indirectly by research. For instance, a series of recent studies have shown that important accomplishments of the preschool and early school years include a decrease in negative emotions, a diminution in the intensity of emotions, and an increase in the use of strategies for managing such emotions. Such research underscores the influence of darker impulses on the toddler and preschool child's experiences, and shows just how it is that children, over time, become more rational and less emotional.

Clinical psychologists have often emphasized the powerful impulses of childhood, and young children's tendency to be dominated by such emotions. Anna Freud famously claimed that if you set a three-year-old to make his way, uncontrolled, from one street corner to another, he would commit every crime in the law books. Implicit in these images, statements, and descriptions—old and new—is the idea that we are born with powerful desires, and little in the way of control mechanisms for reining in those desires.[9] Some researchers have argued that during the early years, fear of punishment is a powerful force in reining in the child's impulsive behavior, whereas older children control themselves with reasoning skills, a more developed awareness of others, and an increased ability to direct themselves toward shared needs and goals.[10] Others have focused on the ways in which children during their second and third years begin to develop ways of inhibiting and controlling their impulses. But even those researchers who have identified early signs of mechanisms such as guilt show that the young child is going through a long, slow process of developing the kinds of control we expect from older children and adults.[11]

Everyday experiences confirm the image of the impulse-driven child. We all know that a two-year-old can have a screaming fit in the middle of a wedding ceremony, and not care one bit about, be in fact completely oblivious to, the irritated or outraged adults around him. While we don't need psychology to point out this kind of behavior (all you need to do is go to the movies), the way we view such behavior, what we think it means about the child, and how we respond to children when they act that way are strongly influenced by our implicit models of early development. In their innovative work characterizing the child-rearing customs in seven different societies, Judy DeLoache and Alma Gottlieb show that many cultures have an implicit belief that you cannot hold very young children responsible for much self-discipline.[12]

Some of the most useful and relevant contemporary research documents the ways in which children learn to rule their impulses rather than be ruled by them. Studies show that most children become increasingly able to delay gratification, to suppress their own needs in observance of shared rules, to redirect their aggression in socially acceptable ways, and to keep certain kinds of pleasure-seeking private. In recent years some studies have focused on individual differences in children's ability to use cognitive strategies for taming their more troublesome impulses. In one study, when children were left alone in a room and admonished not to take a treat that was sitting on a table (they were told that if they could resist, they would get a bigger treat later on), some succeeded by distracting themselves with little songs or games, or even by pretending to sleep. In contrast, other children just kept looking at the cookie or the bell that would signal when the time was up and gave in to temptation sooner. Those children who had been good at using self-distraction to avoid temptation were more sociable and academically successful in school a few years later.[13] The focus on individual differences adds a new dimension to our wild child picture, but nevertheless emphasizes the long-term benefits of taming impulses. A series of intriguing studies has shown that by age seven, children are much more able to talk about their own feelings, and even to reason about the feelings of others.[14] This research adds to our picture of the child who, over time, acquires psychological tools for filtering and cooling the more undiluted emotions of early childhood.

Contemporary research has shown us that self-reflection and self-regulation of emotions are developmental achievements that help a child become socialized and make the child seem less wild. While some philosophers and psychologists have focused on the internal impulses that seem to govern the individual child between the ages of two and five, the wild child metaphor has also shaped our view of children's interactions with others.

Attached to Others

Sigmund Freud and Erik Erikson are famous for describing the long-lasting effects of early experiences of attachment and love. The earliest kind of love emerges, according to Freud, when the baby is nursing. The infant's ability to get enough, to feel fulfilled, and then to extend the basic sensations of feeding to a more complex set of representations and emotions form the cornerstone of the baby's developing emotional life.[15] For Erikson, the baby's first experiences of being cared for determine her basic sense of trust in the social world—"Are my needs met reliably and in a fulfilling way?"[16]

When he toured orphanages during World War II, the British doctor John Bowlby noticed that many babies were only given perfunctory care (changed, fed, and kept safe).[17] The babies were not given any kind of warm or consistent emotional care and attention (the kind a relative or devoted nanny might give). Bowlby noticed that these infants seemed lackluster, wan, and disengaged from the social world. Further, Bowlby argued that there was a link between physical well-being and love. He argued that the babies were suffering physically and developmentally because of the lack of a central emotional relationship and that children who lacked a primary caregiver suffered distinct phases of severe distress. In other words, he argued, children need to feel attached to someone to develop adequately. Hence was born the notion of attachment as a central component of early life, and as a pillar of the developmental process. Meanwhile, the social psychologist Harry Harlow had begun to explore the social attachments of monkeys.[18] He separated infant monkeys from their mothers and raised them in cages that provided them with two kinds of surrogate mothers. One was soft and cuddly but offered no food; the other was wire, but offered a bottle of milk. He found that the baby monkeys preferred to spend their time with the cuddly terrycloth figure. Periodically the baby would scoot over to the wire figure, drink some milk, and then scoot back to the terrycloth figure to cuddle and spend the day. This, he argued, showed that the monkeys' need for comfort and attachment had a more powerful effect on more of their behaviors than did their need for food.

Harlow's research also showed that the nature of this early caregiver arrangement had long-lasting effects on the monkey's social and emotional development. Baby monkeys who were raised without a real monkey as an attachment figure were overly aggressive and maladapted to social life when they reached adulthood.

These views of early life mattered to others besides psychologists. Beginning in the 1930s, psychologists began to convince parents, and to some extent teachers and medical professionals, that young children suffered when they weren't loved. These ideas became refined and extended to show that children's attachment to another person is essential to the child's survival and has long-lasting implications on the child's future relationships, response to authority, and general sense of well-being.

Recent research has shown that certain characteristics of early interactions even affect cognitive skills in later life. Babies who appear to have well-coordinated, sustained interactions with a parent (in which the parent and child look at one another, attune to one another's gaze, vocalize, and make gestures) seem to be more adept at some cognitive skills three years later.[19] This idea, that the kind of attachment a baby forms with others shapes a wide range of experiences and behaviors in later life, grew out of Bowlby's original claims and is most powerfully embodied by one of his protégés, Mary Ainsworth. The conclusions derived from this idea are important, but equally interesting is the way in which it illustrates how observations made of children in real settings can lead to hypotheses that in turn lead to experiments—experiments that take on a life and reality all their own.

Mary Ainsworth reasoned that if attachment is so vital to early well-being, one ought to be able to identify individual differences in the way young children and their mothers relate to one another.[20] Her idea, embodied by the "strange situation paradigm," continues to arouse controversy, generate research, and shape childcare policies. Her work took Bowlby's theory, which focused on the universal nature of attachment, and developed it into a theory of individual differences in attachment style. The basic idea is that a mother and her baby develop a strongly symbiotic attachment during the first year of the baby's life. This attachment provides the toddler with a central base from which to explore the world and develop new relationships. Mothers and their babies have different kinds of attachment. These can be gleaned from watching how mother-child pairs interact. The basic experimental model that Ainsworth invented is ingenious (and problematic). It shows how an insight such as Bowlby's leads to studies of a more precise and contrived nature, which in turn shape years and years of subsequent research and thinking about young children.

Ainsworth's scheme goes like this: A baby and a mother are put in a room together to play. Sometimes another person (a stranger) is in the room and sometimes not. The observer (often looking through a one-way mirror) watches how the mother and her baby play together. Then the mother leaves the room and the observer records the baby's reaction. After a little while the mother reenters the room and the observer watches what the baby does when he is reunited with his mother. One intriguing detail of this research is that the most important piece of evidence comes not from the way the mom and baby play together in the first place, but mostly from how the baby reacts after he is reunited with his mother. Some babies become distraught when their mothers leave the room, but when she comes back they appear overjoyed, giving her a hug, or wrapping themselves around her for a moment. Then they return to their play. Ainsworth categorized these babies as securely attached. Other babies were upset when their mothers left the room, and seemed happy when she returned. But they found it hard to settle back down to play and would keep coming back to interact with their mother, even in negative ways (giving her a smack as if still mad at her for having left). Ainsworth argued that these babies were less able than the securely attached babies to reassure themselves about their mothers, and that their anxiety about her presence (or the possibility of her absence) hampered their play and exploration of the physical environment. A third group of children seemed unconcerned when their mother left the room, and equally unaffected when she returned. Ainsworth terms these children "avoidant."

The debate continues to rage about the validity of Ainsworth's model and its use as a way of determining a child's attachment. Research has shown that children in different cultures deal with the strange situation in ways that reflect cultural habits (whether parents are the primary caregivers, how much closeness is expected between mothers and babies, and so forth). Some research has shown that the way a baby behaves in this experimental setting has little carryover to other situations. Yet on the whole, a vast array of studies has shown that the quality of early attachment has a long-lasting effect on several aspects of the child's later behavior and experience. The dissenting research notwithstanding, most people, in contemporary U.S. society at least, implicitly accept the idea that one's early relationship with one's mother matters. Most significant here, the model emphasizes what human babies have in common with other primates (in Harry Harlow's case the research was with nonhuman primates) and presents the child's primal affective need for attachment as central to her development.

Absorbed by Play

The wild child metaphor has framed our understanding of the infant and toddler's need for attachment as well as her impulse-governed behavior. But its influence goes beyond the realm of the child's emotional life. A great deal of what we have learned about children in recent decades comes from observing and measuring the behaviors that occur when children play. This focus reflects a tacit understanding that there is something distinctive and nonadult-like about the way a child plays as well as what the child plays. Sometimes this playful orientation has been compared to the orientation seen in the youthful play of other species (puppies, primates, and so on). Early childhood educators and psychologists (many of them clinicians) often view play as a primary means through which children explore and express their feelings. Clinicians see children's play as a fairly transparent window onto their fantasies. Children are thought to lack the civilized adult boundaries that keep such fantasies hidden (hence the common therapeutic practice of interpreting children's play, which is assumed to reveal their inner thoughts and impulses). Play, as a predominant mode of expression and of making meaning, is thought to dwindle with age (for instance, we don't expect to see adults begin pretending to be other people, or animals, in the midst of their workday, nor do most therapists expect their adult patients to play in the office as a way of expressing inner thoughts). To some extent our appreciation for the importance of play in childhood has directed us to the child's strong emotions, physical energy, and creativity—their wilder side. But it is also true that by focusing on play we have learned a great deal about how children solve problems and come to think rationally.

Psychologists and parents alike know that the three-year-old can play with a set of blocks for hours on end because of the satisfaction she derives from holding the blocks, moving them around in different patterns, balancing them on top of one another, and possibly even creating structures that allow her to develop various imagined scenarios (this is a barn, and these are all the baby animals). Some of her pleasure, and her deep-seated drive to continue, come from the ways in which her own activity furthers her cognitive development. Building with the blocks, like so many other forms of play, allows her to solve a wide range of cognitive puzzles.

A large body of developmental research over the last one hundred years has shown that whether building a house with blocks, pretending to serve tea using sticks and rocks, drawing pictures in the earth or on paper, or acting out the roles of imagined heroes, children do much of their cognitive "work" by playing. By comparing a wide range of observational and experimental studies, one can see not only that a child's cognitive abilities are at any given point manifested in their play, but also that it is within play that they acquire new cognitive abilities, apply old strategies to new problems, and possibly even encounter the experiences that catapult them to a whole new level of development. Piaget's and Vygotsky's work is filled with accounts of young children developing new mental schema through their encounters with objects and the operations they perform on such objects through play (for instance, children might develop new ways of grouping and categorizing objects by manipulating and sorting them, and in the process discover the principle of equivalence). More recent work on scripts and narratives has shown the ways in which enacting scenarios allows children to develop ideas about sequence and causality. Marjorie Taylor has found that three- and four-year-old children who have imaginary companions have a more sophisticated understanding of how other people think than children who do not have imaginary companions. While her research cannot determine whether such play causes a more sophisticated understanding, research of the kind just mentioned highlights the wide range of cognitive processes that emerge through a child's play.[21]

While these developmental researchers have continued to view the child's powerful impulses, emotional needs, and playfulness as forces to be understood, they also find that such impulses get in the way of research. Researchers often look for an experimental task and setting that will encourage the child to calm down and focus on the activity they want to examine. Parents and teachers are ever eager to find ways to get the child to "settle down" and "learn." Whether we do it implicitly or explicitly, we aim to remove the passionate, unruly, and playful elements in our efforts to civilize, socialize, educate, and investigate the child. Yet we know that these same "wild" elements often drive the acquisition of the cognitive processes that make the child seem more socialized and rational.

Herein lies the crux of an intriguing paradox in developmental research. Huge amounts of empirical and theoretical work, experimental and naturalistic alike, have shown that play forms the bulk of a child's activity, and that within play lies a veritable treasure trove of important and valuable mental processing. Some see play as causing these developments. Others will only allow that play is a crucial context in which such development occurs. But there is little argument that play is a predominant activity within our culture, one in which children become more able, more knowledgeable, and more adult-like. Most or many experiments with young children put them into some kind of play context (with toys, friends, a scenario, or a parent who is instructed to initiate some kind of play, for example). At the same time, more and more of what we have learned about the child's developing mind steers us away from thinking about his playfulness and instead directs our attention toward the highly rational, goal-oriented aspects of his thinking and his development. To take just one measure of this, consider that in the past three years, the top three journals in developmental psychology have published only four articles that focused on play itself. The neglect of play as an important topic for careful descriptive research is in part due to our increasing ability to describe things precisely. The language that psychologists have developed to describe children is beautiful in its clarity and its promise of being able to put into words the subtlest processes and moments of phenomena. With this appetite for precision, however, comes an intolerance of phenomena that are hard to pin down, that are not yet available to finite or contained description. And that brings us to the second metaphor that has pervaded modern thinking about young children—the child as scientist.

THE YOUNG SCIENTIST

Piaget drew an indelible picture of the young child persistently and methodically discovering the way the world works by trying out one operation after another. Here, for instance, he describes his daughter Lucienne in late infancy, watching a matchbox being opened and shut, and a few moments later opening and shutting her mouth.

> L. tries to get a watch chain out of a match box when the box was not more than an eighth of an inch open. She gazed at the box with great attention, then opened and closed her mouth several times in succession, at first only slightly and then wider and wider. It was clear that the child, in her effort to picture to herself the means of enlarging the opening, was using as "signifier" her own mouth, with the movements of which she was familiar tactually and kinesthetically as well as by analogy with the visual image of the mouths of others.[22]

Piaget used this small observation to develop his ideas of how the baby progresses from knowing through action to knowing through thought. He explained that when Lucienne opened and shut her mouth, she was imitating the action of the box. This kind of imitation, he argued, is the first step toward representing events in the mind. By imitating a sequence, Lucienne was making a first effort at representing reality. Moreover, by waiting to imitate it until the event had passed, she showed what he called deferred imitation, the ability to hold onto an image or sequence of events long enough to reenact it without the actual model.

This, he argued, was a crucial step on the path to representational thought, and ultimately the ability to function in abstractions. It is but one example that creates the image of a child fascinated by real-world phenomena. One sees her in an almost silent, uninhabited world, engaged in an endless series of gestures aimed at making sense of how things go together, why sequences unfold in certain ways, and how a certain action leads to a given result.

Just as the wild child view can be found in popular renditions of childhood, so too the view of the child as eager experimenter appears in less scientific, more intuitive constructions of childhood. A. A. Milne, author of *Winnie the Pooh,* captured the same quality of endless fascination with sequences of events and the relationships between objects when he described Eeyore's birthday party. Piglet means to bring a balloon to the party as a gift for Eeyore, but it pops along the way. Pooh means to bring a jar of honey as his gift for Eeyore, but on his way to the party he gets a little hungry and before he knows it, he's eaten all the honey. Once there, all that shamefaced Piglet and Pooh have to offer the guest of honor is a deflated balloon and an empty jar. Eeyore, faced with a deflated balloon and an empty honey jar, discovers that he can put the deflated balloon into the pot, and then take it out again! Thoroughly delighted, he repeats this action over and over again. Eeyore has encountered an inviting puzzle to be solved. Milne wrote his book for children.[23] Much of its enduring appeal is due to the fact that it so often captures interesting characteristics of childhood. Though whimsical, and set in a context in which all kinds of other dynamics are at work, the example brings to life Piaget's view of the young, tireless experimentalist.

What Piaget identified, and Milne intuited, was that children's smallest gestures both reveal and contain their most serious efforts to gain knowledge and to acquire ever more powerful (or more scientific) ways of thinking. This fundamental insight, that children spontaneously and actively try to make sense of their world, predates Piaget. In his classic book *Studies of Childhood,* first published in 1895, James Sully was one of the first (and remains one of the only) to conduct a careful long-term chronicle of young children in their everyday lives. Sully lived in London and was at the center of intellectual life there. He was friends with, among others, Herbert Spencer, Charles Darwin, James Mark Baldwin, and Frances Galton. Like most people working in the field at that time, he was not trained as a psychologist (he was a journalist and later held the post of "chair of mind and logic" at University College, London). But his approach and ideas were molded by those shaping the field of psychology. Sully was interested in providing a detailed description and interpretation of children's minds. Topics he focused on included imagination, aesthetics, morality, and language. He took the approach of a naturalist chronicling a certain species over time in its natural habitat, using descriptions, diary accounts by mothers and nannies, and records kept by teachers to inform his ideas about early development. Indeed, he once said, "Valuable as such statistical investigation undoubtedly is, it is no substitute for the careful methodical study of the individual child."[24] Sully describes the myriad ways in which young children seek to decipher patterns and to make sense of the world around them. Piaget drew on these descriptions in his fundamental insight that children use actions to know the world around them. Piaget's telos was scientific thinking, but like Sully he explored nonlogical forms of thought (for instance, in *The Child's Conception of the World*) as a way of understanding how the child moved toward more logical ways of thinking.[25]

Though Piaget used and amplified Sully's method of close description and interpretation, it was not this methodological aspect of their work that lived on. Instead, Sully's important insight, which Piaget developed into a seminal theory, was that the young child's thought is often thought-in-action. This idea formed a cornerstone of Piaget's work, and provides us still with a powerful tool for illuminating a child's behavior.

Consider a little boy, Ben, sixteen months old and just having learned to walk. He can spend a good while, and a lot of energy, walking around the furniture in his dining room, exploring his own motoric skills as well as the features of the room. But he experiences these features (the hardness and shape of the table legs, for instance) in terms of his own navigations around them (whether his hand will fit around the table leg, for example, if he grasps it). At one point he encounters an empty cardboard box lying on the floor. He lifts a leg to climb into it. But he has underestimated the height of the box side, and his foot bangs against the side of the box. He lifts his leg again, but no higher. In Piaget's terminology, he hasn't yet accommodated to the real features of the box (hasn't changed his schema for the box, which might lead him to lift his leg higher). Finally, on the fourth try, his leg goes up high enough, and he climbs/tumbles inside the box.

The tiniest movements of the young child may contain (and reveal) complex thought processes. As the child grows older, his actions in his environment will become representations about the world, and will lead the child to the discovery of important abstractions about how the world works.

Piaget spent a great deal of his career theorizing about (and attempting to demonstrate) the paths that link early action to more sophisticated forms of thought, especially the mental operations necessary for higher math and science. He argued that through their playful actions, for instance, children learn that a quantity of something doesn't change just because its appearance changes. Piaget's simplest example of this is the young child playing with a small pile of pebbles. Imagine the child setting the pebbles in a straight line. Then the child counts the pebbles. After a while, he moves them around, eventually placing them in the shape of a circle. He counts them again, and sees that he still has the same number of pebbles even though he has changed the shape. He suddenly realizes that the number of pebbles remains the same, no matter what the configuration of the pebbles. Note that he is not learning anything about counting per se, but about the ways in which his actions on the pebbles can and cannot transform them. While this might seem like one tiny discovery among many a child makes over the course of his first twelve years, this particular discovery represents a huge milestone in cognitive development. It represents the idea of conservation of quantity—the idea that a single amount can be contained in different shapes.[26] Why is this important, and why did Piaget single it out? Because it is one example of the kind of understanding that frees human thinkers from the here and now, and from whatever context they are in. Usually the insights that reflect a more pervasive change in the child's thinking are not achieved in a given "aha" moment. Even when they are experienced that way, as in the circle of pebbles example, Piaget and his followers would certainly argue that these moments rest on a long series of encounters with the world. Each encounter leads the child to reorganize what he knows and in some cases to develop new ways of thinking to accommodate new kinds of information that the old ways of thinking won't help him with. As Piaget wrote in his classic book *Biology and Knowledge,* the baby's ability to develop ways of thinking that free him from specific content and specific situations is what releases him from his biological (and possibly evolutionary) constraints.[27]

A vital and predominant piece of what we have learned, and focused on, in the past century of research concerns the child's increasing ability to represent things in her mind, and simultaneously to see beyond appearances, beyond the concrete, to underlying rules, abstractions, and relationships that describe (or constitute) reality as humans know it. From Piaget's perspective, then, two of the most potent discoveries of early mental life are "Things and people are not always as they appear to be" and "Things exist apart from me."

Piaget showed us that children are taken in by whatever is in front of them. In the most well-known illustration of this, if a child looks at two similar balls of clay, she can say with certainty that the balls are the same. If the experimenter rolls one out so that it is long and thin while the other remains a ball, and asks the four-year-old which one is bigger, she will point to the longer one. This is, Piaget claimed, because the child can only think about one dimension at a time (in this case, length) and cannot think past the appearance of the balls to her knowledge that nothing has been added or removed from either ball. The quantity in the clay balls is thus a matter of direct perception, rather than a representation in the child's head. That is, the child is not applying any rules or ideas that are in her head to the idea of the clay. She is simply looking at two globs of clay and notices that one seems longer than the other. Why does this matter? Certainly not because making judgments about quantities or knowing about the principle of conservation of matter comes up as a regular or important feature of a four-year-old's everyday life. The underlying quality of the child's thinking, however, could be pervasive, and indeed is pervasive according to Piagetian thought. It affects everything about the way a four-year-old thinks, solves problems, and experiences her world.

Let me give another example from a somewhat different realm of the child's daily experience. Anyone who has spent a lot of time around a toddler knows that seemingly miraculous moment (or day, or week) when a child utters his or her first real word. Plenty of parents seem to remember forever their first child's first word. My son's was "bridge," which provides a good example of what I want to say about those first words. Typically a child learns a handful of first words, and for some length of time uses the words prodigiously and often for a wide range of purposes. At some point he or she then makes the discovery that everything has a name. It often takes many months to years before she begins to find out that a word is not simply a label for a particular thing, but an abstraction, a sound that represents the idea of something (the word doggie isn't only for her own doggie while it is running to greet her, but for all four-legged furry creatures that bark). In my son's case, bridge was what he said as we passed the George Washington Bridge on our drive into Manhattan. Later he would learn that a bridge is a structure that connects two land masses separated by water. First the name is tied in some way to the object. Quickly thereafter comes the discovery, conscious or otherwise, that everything has a name. That moment of discovery is almost as euphoric and heady for the typical two-year-old as it was for Helen Keller when she learned the word "water." But it is only after weeks or months of learning names of everything that children begin to use and understand that names are the symbolic representations of concepts. The world of things is layered over by a world of symbols. Once they become knowing participants of that world of symbols, children are forever different.

The journey from concrete to abstract thinking is long and complicated, and we still don't know what propels children forward on this path. Do children learn how to represent and abstract? Does someone teach it to them? Do they discover these processes on their own, spontaneously, through their actions? Or do these highly powerful and distinctly human ways of thinking just emerge, the way teeth do, each in their own proper time? While we have not answered all of the questions this view might generate, the sense that development involves increasingly abstract rules and principles still shapes much of what we ask and learn about young children.

Piaget's basic insights continue to determine much of the debate and research in developmental psychology. While much of his specific research has been refuted, expanded, and refined, his basic questions still have a powerful hold on those in the field. Beginning in the early 1970s, however, developmental psychologists began to realize that Piaget's view of the child exploring the world of things on his or her own was missing something important—other people. Psychologists such as Colwyn Trevarthen and Jerome Bruner showed that even the most basic cognitive skills emerge in the context of others. Trevarthen showed that babies eventually learn to contemplate objects with their mothers, literally by looking at an object, looking over at the mother looking at the object, and then looking back at the object again.[28] In the field of social cognition, this was known as social referencing. Jerome Bruner showed that children first learn about the logical sequence of actions by playing games such as peek-a-boo with their mothers.[29] Others such as Michael Cole and Sylvia Scribner showed that what Piaget thought of as mature thinking skills only emerge in cultures where abstraction is used and valued by the community.[30] Eager to find out why adults in Liberia were having such trouble learning math in the new Western school that had been established, Cole and his colleagues began to assess the thinking skills of these Liberians. They found, among other things, that their subjects had difficulty solving syllogisms (a form of logic that requires answering questions based on the relationship between propositions, rather than on the knowledge of the content matter), which were considered an examplar of Piaget's idea of mature cognition. These Liberian subjects lived in a nonliterate community where such abstractions were not valued, nor were they embedded in the everyday learning activities of the culture. Cole and his colleagues demonstrated that what Piaget and his followers thought of as an inevitable and universal achievement was to some extent culturally specific.

Literally hundreds of articles and books have examined the strength and weaknesses of Piaget's model and modified his empirical findings, showing the circumstances under which his conclusions are and are not warranted. In this way the field continues to bear his imprint, through those who have extended his research program and those who have refuted it. Nevertheless, there have been several paradigm shifts that have changed how we think about young children. One of these came about when computers began to pervade our lives.

THE CHILD AS A COMPUTER

One of the great leaps in developmental psychology occurred when a few psychologists began to simulate children's thinking using computers. Artificial intelligence was everywhere in the late 1970s (in fact, the first of only two Nobel Prizes ever given to someone who contributed to psychological research was awarded to Herb Simon for his simulations of thinking using computer models), and people in many fields were eager to see how this amazing new machine could change their work.

For developmental psychologists, the computer as a model had special allure and offered unique advantages. We could set up the kinds of problems children might encounter and see how a computer might go about solving the problem. What information did the computer need to move ahead? In a paper delivered by the developmental psychologist David Klahr in 1982, I got my first real sense of how sensible and helpful it would be to imagine the child as a computer with a set of information, rules, and possible routes to any given solution. He began the paper by telling a story about his son that showed the way in which a child's mind might work something like the flow chart that guided computer processing. He began by saying that one day his son had asked him for the key to the back gate to his house. When Klahr asked why, his son said, "I want to ride my bike!" How, Klahr wondered, did his son get from "I want to ride my bike" to "I need the key to the back gate"? This question led Klahr to speculate that a kind of decision tree had been activated in his son's mind. This decision tree began with a statement of the "Top Goal" (I want to ride my bike) through several conditions and constraints (constraint: I need to wear shoes; condition: my feet are bare) to the final request (ask Daddy for the key to the yard entrance). On first glance this model is appealing because it shows that even those requests and behaviors of young children that seem illogical have an implicit logic to them (such as the conversation Klahr reports at the beginning of his discussion, which goes something like this: "Daddy, would you unlock the basement door?" Daddy: "Why?" Child: "'Cause I want to ride my bike." Daddy: "Your bike is in the garage." Child: "But my socks are in the dryer.").[31] The model, however, goes beyond revealing the internal sense of seemingly childlike non sequiturs. The model suggests that children are capable, under certain circumstances, of thinking in highly organized ways that successfully map out both the real world and a logical system that orders that world, a system that allows the child to operate mentally on the world.

The computer revolution inserted a few powerful ideas into our thinking about young children. One was the notion that much of their thinking was domain specific. Piaget had convinced many that the child's mind goes through pervasive structural changes that underlie all kinds of specific changes in functioning. In Piaget's view, the four-year-old, not yet able to think about his representations of objects and the relations between those representations, solves problems in one way. A ten-year-old, by contrast, who has begun to think about the rules and logic that govern objects, will solve problems in a completely different way from the four-year-old. According to Piaget, if you give a four-year-old some blocks and ask him to group them or count them in a certain way, you can predict how he will perform the task or solve the problem based on what you know about his overall level of development. This is so, according to Piaget, because almost all tasks are going to draw on the same structural qualities that define a child of that particular age. The beauty of this idea was that it was simple (each age was defined by a stage, and each stage could, supposedly, predict how a child would function under a wide range of conditions). The child seemed consistent, and similar to others his or her age, and the theory thus suggested, implicitly, that specific experiences didn't matter that much. As long as children had some interactions with objects and events (mostly natural events) in the world, their way of thinking would move from one level to another, regardless of which materials they encountered, what kinds of tasks they confronted, and what activities filled their day.

The computer model, on the other hand, implied a different developmental path. Psychologists such as David Klahr, Jean Mandler, Micheline Chi, and Roger Schank used this model to argue that, like computers, children extracted information from their environment and used that information to build rules and modify future actions (the way a computer does).[32] Each encounter with a certain set of information or materials affected the child's knowledge and expectations about a given domain. In other words, experience mattered, and not just as a general kind of fuel for the engine. Instead whatever set of problems and materials one engaged with regularly would lead to a more advanced set of solutions and strategies in that domain, and might make the child more developmentally advanced than he was in some other domain. This meant that children had to know about a topic in order to think at a higher level within that domain. Micheline Chi, for instance, showed that children who were top chess players had much better memory for new chess positions than children who were not chess players.

Why is this finding and its implications important? Because it suggests that expertise rather than some general way of thinking determines how a person will solve a problem, or how well they will "think" in a given domain. The computer model also led us to consider the possibility that development is more continuous than Piaget and the other developmentalists from the early part of the century had suggested. That is, a child develops increasingly sophisticated strategies bit by bit as he takes in new experiences and knowledge, rather than undergoing some across-the-board pervasive reorganization at certain critical junctures. One striking implication of the computer model was the idea that children are not all that different from adults in the way they think. The young child encountering a new domain (say, chess) does the same thing, to some extent, that the adult would: modify her strategies and expectations as she has new experiences within the domain. This has fed the incipient notion, described in Chapter 1, that children are simply smaller or incomplete adults. Though the failure to take full stock of the qualitative differences between the child and the adult mind can be traced to several sources, the model of information processing is certainly one of those sources.

The most exciting outcome of the computer zeitgeist was the idea that early on children recognize and internalize the basic outlines of everyday experiences—they form "scripts" of routine events. This notion began with the influential book *Scripts, Plans, and Goals,* written by Roger Schank and Robert Abelson, two psychologists who worked with the artificial intelligence model.[33] They argued that people experience everyday life in terms of scripts that have people, places, and actions, and that most often these scripts are organized around meaningful goals (the "go to work" script, the "family gathering" script, and so forth). The developmental psychologist Katherine Nelson used this work as a springboard for a new way of thinking about how children's thinking develops in the first five years of life. She argued that children quickly and easily get hold of daily experience by detecting the underlying scripts that shape and guide daily life.[34] She reasoned that in the first years of life children experience a series of routines (breakfast, going to day care, or going to the park, for instance) that offer them a set of maps, that tell them what to expect. These maps are organized, as Schank and Abelson had argued, around goals involving actors and actions unfolding in a particular time and place. Unlike the Piagetian notion, Nelson's paradigm suggested that children's understanding of how the world works (including such complex aspects of knowledge as concepts and language) grew out of their everyday encounters with a world full of people and events, rather than simply solitary interactions with objects.

Nelson's initial research along these lines was remarkable in its seeming simplicity and its influence on our thinking. She found that asking children what they ate for breakfast that morning left most three-year-olds shrugging and looking blankly back at the experimenter. But when asked, "What do you usually eat for breakfast?" they could offer a clear, and by and large accurate, script of what breakfast time entails (first we have juice, then we have toast, then sometimes we eat bacon, then mommy puts my shoes on, and we are done). These scripts suggested that when children are as young as three they have formed mental models of how their daily experiences are organized. Moreover, these models include certain core features: events are set in time and place, and follow a logical order.

Nelson's work had a tremendous effect on the field of child psychology. It made children seem much smarter and more able to sort things out than previous research had suggested. It also provided us with an alternative route to children's intellectual development. Sophisticated ways of thinking did not come from small experiments on the world that led to increasingly powerful theories (the child as emerging scientist); instead the child's "higher order" thinking emerged out of his or her understanding of everyday life. This shift, from assuming that children extracted scientific principles about the world from their encounters with objects, to the view that children used everyday, real-world sequences to order their thoughts, was a dramatic one. It visualized the child in a world of people and activities, rather than alone in a room with objects. It suggested that children know more than research had shown, and that often the problem was one of knowing how to "get at" the child's real abilities (asking "what happens" elicited greater capabilities than asking "what happened").

Over time, Nelson shifted her view somewhat. Early on, one got the sense from her descriptions and studies that children just naturally detected the script-like structure of everyday events, and used these as a basis for other kinds of thinking (concept development, for instance). But as the theory evolved, Nelson placed more and more emphasis on the mediated nature of scripts. Scripts don't, she concluded, simply exist in the world, or in the child's mind, but are the socially meaningful forms that children use to order their world. While children everywhere may use scripts to make sense of experience, and develop more abstract and complex ways of thinking as they get older, the child acquires these scripts through interactions with others (parents, teachers, and friends) and the scripts themselves bear the flavor of local customs.

Nelson's work paved the way for a tidal wave of research aimed at identifying when and how children form scripts for everyday experiences, and to understanding the ways in which those scripts might provide children with building blocks for other kinds of intellectual achievements. For instance, scripts might provide children with a framework within which to create specific memories for unique events. It was thought that children had little ability to recall specific events in any coherent form. But script theory gave us a way of seeing how the child might make her way from a general outline of a type of event (going to day care) to a specific narrative of some special version of the event (the time we got to day care and it was all black and the electricity was off). In one ingenious study, Katherine Nelson and Joan Lucariello found that children were more able to develop conceptual categories for things they had first learned about through scripts. They offered three-year-olds two different kinds of experiences with the same objects—for instance, toy animals. In one version children were allowed to play and group the animals according to category (lions, elephants, and so on). In another version they participated in script-like enactments involving the animals (all the things that happened at a circus). When asked later to name members of conceptual groups, they were much more likely to be able to do so in the context of questions about script-like experiences (all the animals in a certain circus act).[35] The idea pervading this research was that well-known events, and their mental representation, gave children a basis for all kinds of mental work. It stressed two related principles: That children's intellect develops through their encounters with the socially mediated world of people doing things in places, and that scripts, or representations of these experiences, are more central to mental development than are more abstract principles that govern the natural world.

THE SYMBOL-USING SOCIAL CHILD

The recognition that other people play a central role in children's development did not begin with information processing or with Katherine Nelson, but dates as far back as the beginning of the twentieth century, in Russia. While Piaget was watching and interviewing children in Geneva, a young genius named Lev Vygotsky was conducting a wide range of studies in the young Soviet Union.[36] Though a contemporary of Piaget's, his work only entered the mainstream of psychology in the late 1980s, partly through the research and writings of people such as Nelson. Thus while a chronological account would place him with Piaget, an intellectual history puts him much later, when he began to have a strong influence on other researchers.

Among Vygotsky's most famous and influential contributions to developmental psychology was his demonstration that from very early on in the child's life, her development is shaped by those around her. Specifically, Vygotsky argued that the tools and symbols we use to work with and to think with shape our thoughts—and that these tools and symbols are profoundly influenced by the values, modes of thinking, and customs of our culture and community.

There were two specific and potent implications to this aspect of Vygotsky's work. One was the idea that what children do with other people foreshadows what they will be able to do on their own at a later date. Though overused and oversimplified in recent years, the core of this idea is rich and generative. It suggests that many cognitive skills first unfold with other people, in a kind of dialogue of action. Part of development, then, consists of the process by which these collaborative activities are internalized by the child and eventually become part of the child's internal mental repertoire. This has huge implications for our model of development, suggesting as it does that looking at pairs or groups of people is as important a window on cognitive activity as looking at the individual.

The second implication concerns the power of mediation. Tools, as well as symbols (such as words) are the means by which shared interpretations, meanings, values, and solutions become part of a person's inner life. As the child internalizes strategies and skills first learned with others, she also internalizes a way of thinking. Not only other people, but also the symbols and tools shared by people, become central to the child's mental life. In other words, as the child takes in her culture, her mind is to some extent shaped by those mental processes first learned with others. In addition, an intriguing and often overlooked aspect of his work was his understanding that though these culturally shared symbols might influence one's inner thought processes, there remained some aspects of thinking beyond the realm of socialized thought—that is, the inner life is never fully shaped by others.

Some of Vygotsky's most wonderful studies involved recording the ways in which young children's language guides their actions as they solve problems. Nelson's work, too, though it was originally sparked by discoveries made in information processing, drew increasingly on the ideas of Vygotsky and his focus on the role of mediation in the development of thought. The tendency of young children to narrate and guide their problem solving, which Vygotsky first documented, leads us to the next great insight in developmental psychology.

Becoming Reflective

If symbol use and the abstract thinking it leads to cause a revolution in the child's mental life, then another, albeit gradual, revolution occurs as the child becomes reflective. In a pivotal article, written in the early 1980s, the late Ann Brown changed the way we thought about what exactly it is that develops in children's thinking.[37] Brown was interested in memory and why children seem to get better at remembering things as they get older. Prior to her work there had been two prevailing explanations for why children's memory improved with age. Most people had assumed the improvement in memory ability was simply a matter of capacity—that an increase in memory capacity was a maturational process, and did not depend on specific kinds of learning or practice. Piaget, by contrast, argued that the reason older children are better at remembering than younger children is that as they become more able to represent reality rather than simply interact with it directly, and as they begin to apply more abstractions to those representations (thinking in terms of relations, rules, and concepts), they can use such mechanisms to aid their memory, which in turn expands their capacity. In other words, he thought that memory improvement was the result of underlying changes in cognitive capacity.

Imagine you have presented a child with a tray on which you have placed an array of objects: a toy car, a crayon, a doll, a pair of scissors, a banana, a pencil, a toy tea cup, an apple, and a piece of candy. You show them to the child for a few minutes. Then you take them away, and a few minutes later ask the child to name all of the things he saw. A three-year-old is likely to answer you quickly and to recall perhaps two of the items. By the time a child is six years old, however, he will be able to remember most if not all of the items. What has changed? People used to assume that a child's memory capacity simply got larger, the way his muscles get bigger. Piaget argued that in fact an important cognitive change takes place that accounts for the improvement in memory tasks. He said that the crucial development is the child's ability to mentally represent objects in conceptual groups. This ability to think about things in terms of abstract concepts (foods, toys, or tools in the earlier example), according to Piaget, accounts for a general shift in the way the child represents and thinks about the world. For many years after Piaget demonstrated this, psychologists (and educators) assumed that the acquisition and use of concepts ("pre-operational thought," in Piaget's terminology) explained memory behavior.

What Ann Brown argued, however, was strikingly different, and added a whole new facet to what we think of as development. She said that it is the process of monitoring your own memory activity—thinking about thinking, in other words—that changes during childhood. The four-year-old just does what he does, whereas the six-year-old thinks about how best to help himself remember, uses mnemonics, and is deliberate in his efforts to remember. This idea extends far beyond a memory task involving objects on a tray. It implies that one of the key changes during the first twelve years of life is the child's ability to reflect on his or her own thought processes, and that this reflectiveness dramatically expands the child's problem-solving abilities.

For a long time, the work of Ann Brown and others led us to focus on the child's ability to think (and be able to talk) about her own cognitive processes, and to view such awareness as a sign of the child's growing competence. Paradoxically, recent research has demonstrated that it is quite common for young children to develop new strategies for problem solving at an implicit level before they develop any awareness (or reflectiveness) about how they are solving the problem. So on the one hand we have an increasingly reflective self-conscious problem solver (the scientist monitoring his own methods), and on the other hand, a problem solver who often intuits a solution before she even knows she is doing so (the scientist's "aha" moment).

Robert Siegler is a developmental psychologist who has long been interested in identifying, step by step, the ways in which children think through various cognitive problems. Recently he has become interested in the kinds of insights children might have when trying to solve problems, particularly insights of which they may be unaware.[38]

Even adults often have trouble knowing—and communicating about—how they learn something new, or how they figure out a new solution. But with a child the process is far more mysterious. Siegler reasoned that with some kinds of numerical puzzles, one could solve the problem step by step, whereas if one were to figure out a rule, it would make solving the problem much quicker. For instance, if you take the sum of two numbers minus the second number, the answer will always be the first number ($2 + 3 - 3 = 2$). The mathematical principle at work ($a + b - b = a$) may seem obvious or self-evident to any adult reading this book, but for the child of seven the underlying principle is not obvious. A typical child sitting down to solve the problem $5 + 2 - 2$, for example, might reasonably follow through on a sequence of simple calculations:

> The child would first add 5 to 2 and get 7
> Then the child would subtract 2 from 7 and get 5
> Finally, the child would know that the answer is 5.

Siegler reasoned that at some point most children figure out the underlying rule (that $a + b - b = a$). Once a child has identified the underlying principle, they no longer spend the time doing the sequence of actual calculations; instead, as soon as the children recognize the type of problem it is, they know the answer is the number that they started with. Thus, Siegler reasoned, a child using the principle to answer the question would spend less time on one of these problems than a child who has not discovered the principle and is still doing the calculations.

When Siegler gave these problems to children to solve, he found that by the time they are seven they almost always get the right answer. But they begin solving them faster several problems before they actually articulate the rule they are using. In other words, children use the principle before they are aware of the principle. Siegler argues that this is evidence that children use insights about problems before they become aware of and are able to articulate their insights. Siegler has found a way to reveal a process that the subject doesn't even yet know he is using.

Perhaps children discover rules and principles before they can be reflective about them. This would suggest that children need a chance to work on problems and discover solutions and formulas without necessarily learning the rule explicitly—and that more learning takes place implicitly and in context than many school practices would indicate. Adults have tended to assume that if children can explain something they can understand it, and that if they can't explain it they can't understand it. But it turns out that understanding often emerges in two stages, first an implicit one and then an explicit one. The implicit and thus more invisible kind of understanding may often be a prerequisite for the more explicit kind of understanding. More fundamentally, this elegant line of research has helped developmental psychologists adjust our model of cognitive development. Much of what goes into a pervasive shift in thinking occurs in small fits and starts within specific contexts. Often those fits and starts are invisible to actor and observer alike.

The child Siegler imagines is only sometimes reflective and able to describe his own strategies and cognitive processes. Blending this view with that of Brown's child, someone whose skills are enormously enhanced by the ability to be reflective, gives us a more variegated view of the child solving problems. It stills leaves us, however, with a strangely asocial child.

LITTLE PSYCHOLOGISTS

One problem that has haunted cognitive psychologists (Piagetians and artificial intelligence theorists alike) has been their tendency to portray children as lone actors in a confusing world that demands order. With Piaget the order seemed to be found at a deep and abstract level. Quantities of clay, three-dimensional scenes, and pebbles elicited understanding from the child. Meanwhile, those interested in scripts and other information-processing models emphasized a world filled with people and events. The child was led to connect physical reality to social reality. One imagines a child entering a situation (a birthday party, for instance) and detecting patterns (first we open presents, then we play a game, then we eat cake) as the scene unfolds. Wild child theorists, at the same time, have tended to think of the child as being unconcerned with how others feel and act (apart from how other people make them feel or fulfill their needs). This has left the field with a puzzle or two. First of all, imagine a three-year-old sitting in her room with her mother, and saying to her mother, "You be mommy bear. I'm baby bear. When I say, 'I'm hungry,' you feed me this apple." The mommy dutifully sits there, doing nothing differently, and yet somehow fulfilling the role of mommy bear. At some point, the little girl says in a high squeaky voice, "I'm hungry." And if the mother is correctly following orders, she then hands baby bear a pretend apple (a piece of felt). Why is the little girl not surprised that her mother is treating a piece of felt as if it were an apple? How does she know that her mother is pretending? Would she be surprised if her mother actually started chewing on the felt? The answer is that she "knows" in one way or another that her mother, like her, is pretending.

In our culture at least, encounters such as these are such a regular part of everyday life that we rarely notice that they involve complex psychological maneuvers on the part of the child. But in recent years, psychologists have recognized that these moments contain a vital kernel of human adult thinking—the ability to think about the thoughts of other people. Psychologists have come to realize that human beings do something other species do not, which is to develop ideas and hypotheses about our own thought processes, and to use these ideas and hypotheses to think about the thoughts and intentions of others. The ability to speculate on other people's intentions, beliefs, and thoughts—what many have come to call our folk psychology—provides us with an incredibly powerful tool for navigating through life.

But if this skill is so central, when and how do we begin using it?

Playing with pebbles won't give it to us, and neither will mapping the usual sequence of events. Neither of these directly involves interpretations of people's behaviors, facial expressions, and words. Neither the wild child, the scientist, nor the robot quite captures what many parents and teachers intuitively know, which is that the child often displays an uncanny sense of why other people are behaving in a certain way.

To some psychologists during the 1980s and 1990s it became clear that there was something going on in the minds of young children that went beyond the kinds of logical relations that Piaget attended to, or the kinds of everyday order on which script theory focused. For instance, when David Klahr's son asked him for the key to the back gate, and explained the request by saying "Because my socks are in the dryer," his thoughts probably were focused not only on questions of logical necessity. He must have also been thinking about his father: what he might say yes or no to and what kind of answer might or might not satisfy his father's probing. As psychologist Dennis Newman (among others) pointed out in his work on children's mathematical problem solving in school settings, even when children are struggling with tasks as decontextualized as school math, they often succeed or fail based on how well they read the intentions, habits, and demands of the people around them.[39]

We needed to get a better understanding of how and when children first come to construct and use insights about other people's thoughts and intentions. This has come to be known as theory of mind. The idea is that we all develop a theory of mind, a set of expectations and beliefs about what other people will think. Research has shown that we begin life without an awareness, understanding, or sensitivity to the thoughts and intentions of others. The two-year-old does not seem to know that other people may walk into a room or situation and see things from a different perspective than he does. Piaget first described this as egocentrism. He argued that children think everyone experiences the world from their own particular vantage point. Preschool teachers see this when a two-year-old "reads" a book to others—invariably she makes no effort to show the other children what she alone sees on the page, thinking that everyone can already see it because she can. Though researchers such as Margaret Donaldson have shown that Piaget underestimated the child's ability to think about other perspectives (for instance with her "cookie thief" experiment described in Chapter 1), only in the past ten years or so have psychologists honed in on the significance of the child's burgeoning ability to think about other people's thoughts.[40] Until recently, critics of the egocentric view of toddlers and preschoolers have rather narrowly focused on identifying the conditions under which children were able to take another's perspective. To their credit, this research has given us a more finely tuned picture of the child's perspective-taking ability. A child who might have failed Piaget's three-mountain task, for instance, can solve a similar problem when given a sensible story within which the other person's perspective is useful and interesting.

But theory-of-mind research has gone beyond this paradigm to suggest that within the first five years young children develop at least a rudimentary set of principles or rules that help them figure out what another person might think in a given situation. For instance, Daniella O'Neill has shown that when faced with an appealing toy placed on a high shelf, a two-year-old child's gestures will vary as a function of whether the mother was present when the toy was put out of reach.[41] This suggests that even at two children have some rudimentary sense of what the other person does and does not know.

One of the most vivid examples of this kind of thinking occurs when a person has to reckon with the fact that another individual may have different thoughts and intentions than his own. Examples that force us to make a distinction between our thoughts and the thoughts of others abound, even in the experiences of young children. For instance, a child who hides a toy from a friend must have some idea that he knows something the friend does not know. This distinction can be found in many children's stories as well. At some point a child, hearing "Little Red Riding Hood" read aloud, must realize that though she knows it is the wolf lying in Granny's bed, Little Red Riding Hood mistakenly believes it to be Granny.[42] Once researchers began to realize that the capacity to think about the thoughts and beliefs of others as separate from one's own thoughts and beliefs represents a pivotal developmental shift, they faced an intriguing challenge. They needed to devise a method for finding out what children think about other people's beliefs and thoughts.

The most famous (and clever) method to investigate what children know and think about other people's intentions and thoughts involves what is called a "false belief"—that is, it explores how a child predicts that another person's actions will depend on information that person has, even if the child knows more or different information. In other words, when does the young child know that Little Red Riding Hood doesn't know that the wolf is in the house, even though the reader knows it, and that therefore Little Red Riding Hood will go inside? One important assumption of this line of thinking is that the child develops an overall theory about how people's minds affect their actions—thus each insight does not stem from specific intuitions about a given situation, but expresses an emerging "theory."

In one of the most famous false belief experiments, the researcher Joseph Perner constructed a story about a little boy named Maxi.[43] Maxi's mother has just come in from shopping and Maxi is helping her unload the groceries. He finds a chocolate bar and puts it into a drawer so that he can eat it later. Then he goes out to play. While he is out, his mother finds the chocolate bar in the drawer and moves it to the cupboard with her other baking ingredients. The question for the child participating in the experiment is: When Maxi comes back in, where will he look for the chocolate bar? Children under three answer that Maxi will look in the cupboard. They cannot distinguish between what they know and what the character knows.

By the time children are five years old, however, most seem able to figure out that Maxi doesn't know what they know, and that he will probably look first in the last place he saw the chocolate. Maxi has what is known as a false belief (his belief is based on incomplete information). What is intriguing is not only the way in which researchers figured out how to test this change in how children think about other people's thoughts, but also the seeming universality of the findings. No matter how one tinkers with the experiment, and all kinds of permutations and modifications have been tried, before age four few kids solve the puzzle, and by age five most kids solve it easily. Perner's Maxi story and Siegler's mathematical experiment are but two illustrations of the wealth of research done over the past fifty years that critiques, refutes, extends, and reinvents the kinds of things Piaget first noticed at the beginning of the twentieth century.

The work on theory of mind and false beliefs exemplifies the great methodological and empirical progress that has occurred in the last five decades. But some of the studies within this paradigm also manifest an interesting and, to my mind, disturbing trend in the way we think about young children. Paradoxically, some of the theory-of-mind work, which often has used stories and other play-like activities (such as hiding M & M candies from puppets), has bypassed or overlooked the child's playfulness. That is, some of this research has perpetuated our tendency to undervalue the significance of the child's playful modes of thought, and overestimated the child's tendency to approach problems in a purely rational, deliberative manner even for tasks that might seem to invite play. I believe that playfulness, as opposed to play, may permeate some of the seemingly most rational problems of all. At the same time, certain kinds of thinking that emerge in play, and entailing a playful orientation, may be the precursors to more rational forms of thinking.

Paul Harris has an interesting view of how sophisticated logical forms of thought may be rooted in child's play. He has argued that Piaget treated play as a kind of primary or immature form of thought, one in which reality was subsumed by fantasy in order to serve the child's wishes and primitive needs. This formulation, according to Harris, stemmed in part from Freud's view that primary process thinking (the kind found in dreams and possibly in imaginary play) was developmentally prior to secondary process thinking. But, Harris argues, in fact play and imaginative thinking are essential to what we take as highly developed mature forms of thinking (problem solving, imagining alternative outcomes, envisioning beyond the here and now, and so forth). Harris argues that the kinds of thinking involved in play and imaginative "work," as he calls it, are not different from those used in rational thought, and that in fact the ability to imagine, transform reality, and construct worlds with symbols constitutes our highest intellectual abilities.

> The particular evolutionary path taken by modern Homo sapiens was marked not just by the emergence of complex language or the ability to conjure up situations in the imagination. Rather, at some point in our evolutionary history, there was an explosive fusion of these two capacities. That fusion of language and imagination would have enabled us to pursue a new type of dialogue—to exchange and accumulate thoughts about a host of situations, none actually witnessed but all imaginable: the distant past and future, as well as the magical and the impossible.[44]

In a recent line of research meant to explore this idea, Harris and some of his colleagues asked children to respond to stories that contain what they call counterfactuals—possibilities for rethinking a story in terms of a different cause and effect. In one study, Harris and Robert Kavanaugh asked children between the ages of three-and-a-half and six-and-a-half to answer questions about stories that involved these counterfactuals. In one version, for instance, the experimenter says, "Cathy wanted something to eat. Her Mom said she could have a big cookie or a little cookie. Cathy chose a big cookie. Afterwards she felt nice and full. Why did she feel nice and full?" Clearly one possible way for a child to think this through is to imagine what would have happened if Cathy had eaten the small cookie. The researchers are interested in when and how children come to be able to think of a sequence of events that runs counter to the way they have happened. They found that even their youngest subjects could draw on counterfactual reasoning.[45]

Harris demonstrates, quite elegantly, how children think within an imaginary framework, and shows that very young children can engage in sophisticated and complex kinds of reasoning within a fictional or play framework. One fascinating piece of evidence he uses to support his view of children's imaginative thinking is his argument that children with autism, far from being stuck in a fictive world as often thought, have a great deal of difficulty playing imaginatively at all. He uses this to convince us that imagination and playful thought processes are not primitive (or to use Piaget's term, autistic). Instead, Harris argues, imagination is developmentally advanced. Moreover, the lack of it is a good indicator that a child has developmental problems.

Harris draws a line of continuity between the fictive world the young child creates and the fictive worlds that adults either enter into (say, by reading a novel) or create (perhaps by writing a novel). His work moves the theory-of-mind paradigm ahead by showing us that when a child makes up a scenario, either with play gestures or with language, she engages in a powerful form of thinking. Imagining alternatives (and articulating them, in words or gestures), transforming objects, manipulating symbols, and thinking about the dual status of a symbol or object are some of the most potent tools we have for thinking through ideas and problems as adults. Can the three-, four-, or five-year-old think about what might have happened in a given scenario, and reimagine things according to a different set of facts? The idea here is that what might seem like an esoteric skill rarely used in everyday life is both the stuff of play and the stuff of sophisticated adult thinking. For instance, take the familiar example of a couple of children in a dress-up area pretending to be mommies and daddies. Much of their play will involve mirroring events they have seen and experienced in their own kitchen or perhaps observed, for instance by watching television. But the children also transform events and people through their enactments. So the mommy now not only offers to cook pizza, but also will serve several chocolate cakes. The daddy will not marry just the one mommy; he will marry two mommies. These small transformations are essential not only for what they tell us about a child's specific concerns, images, and experiences, but also because they are a manifestation of the essential human activity of transforming reality and thinking about things not as they are, but as they might be.

The stories used in most studies of counterfactual thinking, however, are unlikely to elicit children's most engaged thinking processes because they are quite different from the kinds of stories and scenarios that typically grab the attention of young children. As mentioned earlier in this chapter, some research has shown that using emotionally charged material sometimes elicits higher levels of cognitive processing than more neutral material. Often children respond to the tension or drama of a story (someone got in trouble) and can find it difficult to shift their focus away from the "hot" aspect of the story to a "cool" aspect (it's difficult to stop thinking about the trouble and start thinking of logical alternatives).

In fact we have some evidence that a child's cognitive skills are often enhanced when their deeper passions are engaged. In studying children's attachment by asking children questions about stories, psychologist Inge Bretherton found that when she used stories that described a dispute among family members, her three-year-old subjects gave much richer responses than had been given in studies using less emotionally charged material.[46] It would be useful to look at children's logic about various kinds of experience (pretense, narrative, hypothetical situations, and everyday events) in ways that take their emotional priorities into account. Feeling seems to be an inextricable part of the development of thinking. Judy Dunn, for example, found that thirty-three-month-old children who engaged in more talk about emotions at home (discussions of sibling disputes, for instance) performed better on theory-of-mind tasks (such as the Maxi task) at forty months.[47]

While Harris has made a compelling case for the idea that adults and children alike enter fictive worlds, and think in complex rational, logical ways within those worlds, he doesn't show the flip side, which is that there is something qualitatively distinct about the way children, as opposed to adults, experience the movement back and forth between the fictive and factual worlds. In other words, there are two crucial pieces missing from this particular puzzle, and they may be connected to one another. First, a full understanding of children's pretense will have to include a more precise and full description of the ways in which children experience pretense (as opposed to how they perform on pretense tasks). When are they excited by what they play, and when does play fulfill some kind of soothing, calming function? When does the pretend versus nonpretend distinction seem salient and relevant to young players and when is it unimportant? What themes and forms of play are most compelling to children, and is there any pattern to what interests children of certain ages, developmental stages, or personalities? These are just a few examples of the kinds of questions that need to be addressed. Second, how exactly do children move back and forth between pretense and nonpretense? Children's solutions and strategies may be similar in the imaginary and everyday domains, but that does not necessarily mean that the experience of thinking and functioning within those two realms is similar. Characterizing such experience is essential if we are ever to know what it is about childhood that is different from adulthood.

Knowing how to make someone turn out smart, or productive, or sane, is extremely important. To find out these things one has to measure behavior and trace influences. But as I argued in Chapter 1, there are other reasons for studying young children. If we want to understand childhood for its own sake, measuring outcomes is not as useful as trying to get the fullest picture possible of what children do and what they experience as they do it. In order to have a full understanding of children's pretense, we need to find out how it feels to construct and enter a fictive world, and how the world looks from within that fictive world. Let me illustrate this point with a story about a four-year-old boy, Charlie. He was playing with his mother outside, and he said to her, "Let's pretend that you are the mommy and I am your little boy." She responded, "But I AM your mommy, and you ARE my little boy." He responded, "Yes, but let's just PLAY that, okay?" The point is that Charlie, like many children, took an "as if" stance toward reality—different from the everyday orientation used to dig in the sandbox, empty out a backpack, or pick out a splinter. Harris makes the point that once having taken that stance, the child can think in a way that is analogous to the analytic modes we usually ascribe to older, schooled children. What the story about Charlie reminds us, however, is that the act of taking that stance, the boundary between fictive and nonfictive, is just as important as the kind of thinking he engages in within the frame. Vygotsky discussed just this kind of boundary crossing when he described two young sisters pretending to be sisters. While adults may too cross boundaries and switch frames, it seems to be an important aspect of childhood that has received far too little attention.

While Harris has made an important link between the imaginative work of the young child and the imaginative work of the adult, and shown us the rule-governed sense of the child's transformations, Nelson has been arguing that the root of these transformations is somewhat different than we first thought. Early theory-of-mind researchers like Joseph Perner and Henry Wellman found that the three-year-old could not solve problems like the hidden M & M's, and four-year-olds could. They attributed the change to a shift in the child's logical abilities. The four-year-old can figure out that the puppet doesn't know where to look for the M & M's because the puppet needs information it doesn't have in order to look in the right place. This perspective is based, so Perner and Wellman speculated, on the child's newfound ability to understand the logical connection between facts and knowledge, or knowledge and beliefs, and to keep clearly in his mind the difference between his own knowledge and that of someone with different information.[48] In recent years, however, Nelson has argued that whereas children older than four can solve problems like the M & M problem or the Maxi problem, this ability does not emerge out of some logical blueprint that they automatically acquire or mature into at about age four. In a provocative study, Nelson and a graduate student gave the Maxi stories to adults. While of course almost all of the adults could answer the false belief question correctly, their reasons varied in interesting ways. While some gave classic logical answers (Maxi would look in the last place he saw the chocolate because he can't know what happened after he left the room), many gave what Nelson called "narrative" or "interpretive" answers.[49] These adults might offer some analogy from their own experience (I was always hiding the baking stuff from my kids when they were little. I had to be really sneaky about where to put it), or embellish the Maxi scenario as they explained it. Nelson argued that this provided evidence for a different developmental route to the theory of mind. She argues that rather than developing a set of logical rules that enable the child to correctly answer questions about the Maxi story, children draw on their narrative encounters with the world to reason about other people—to determine what others know, believe, and do. In other words, the young child is not answering questions about other people's intentions based on an acquired set of logical rules (for example, a person won't look for something in a drawer if he doesn't know it's there), but rather draws on recollections (narratives) of previous experiences with people (he'll look where he last saw it because last time I lost something, I looked for it where I had last seen it).

Nelson's work reminds us that the child doesn't need a theory of mind before she can interpret the minds of other people. What she needs is experiences with others, and her natural inclination to understand those experiences in a narrative framework. Out of those encounters comes a more formal set of rules and interpretations. Nelson makes a compelling analogy when she argues for the idea that narrative experience comes first, and logical rules, second. Romans built amazing bridges long before science had discovered or articulated the physics of suspension and support. One can build a bridge without a theory of bridges. In the same way, the child can understand the thoughts and intentions of others without a theory about thoughts and intentions.

Taken together, Harris and Nelson have provided two very important advances in our understanding of how children come to think about the thoughts of others. Harris has shown the kinds of thinking that are inherent in imaginary play, and demonstrated how closely linked they are to the kinds of thinking highly valued in adult life. Nelson has provided evidence that these kinds of thinking emerge from real experiences and narrative forms of those experiences. In that way she has put the thinking, feeling, acting child back into the scenario. But as developmental psychologist Margery Franklin said when reviewing this literature, Nelson's depiction of early development leaves us with an "irredeemably sensible child."[50] Franklin's comment refers to Nelson's emphasis on the child's attention to, and urge to make useful sense of, everyday situations. Her examples show children drawing on fairly ordinary real-life scenarios, and there is little mention of the imagined and sometimes fantastical inner dramas that might also influence a child's interpretation of experience. Though Nelson's view of how the theory of mind develops is less abstract and more real than those that came before, the child is still treating problems as texts to be interpreted—that is, acting in a hyper-rational, cool way, rather than in the hotter, more fluid ways in which children often can be seen responding to situations. Nelson's view of how children begin to interpret and solve problems in everyday experience may tell part of the developmental story, but it does not capture the living, breathing child well enough.

LOOKING AHEAD

This brings me to the interesting problem posed by developmental psychology. More and more, psychologists begin with a theory, and then try to find behaviors in children that will support or refute that theory. Take, for example, Katherine Nelson's research on children's accounts of their day. Nelson theorized that children learn about the general form of experience before they develop memories for specific experiences. This led her to modify the previous research, in which experimenters asked children "What did you eat for breakfast this morning?" to instead ask, "What do you usually eat for breakfast?" As we have seen, this led to important findings about what three- and four-year-olds could do. They can answer general questions, even when they cannot answer the specific (they know what they usually do, even when they aren't at all sure what they did that very morning). But this change in tactic also demonstrates the way in which the theory determines the research, which in turn determines, to some extent, what one can see in the child. Note that if she had said, "Let's play breakfast" she might have elicited a more complex representation of breakfast routines, one less skeletal and more permeated with specific information, or even perhaps including imaginary information. In another example, when researchers Nancy Stein and Tom Trabasso elicited stories from young children to test their ability to organize events in a logical sequence, they found that five-year-olds cannot sequence logically and eight-year-olds can.[51] But the theory that drove the research precluded discovering that logical order was not relevant to young children's storytelling impulses.

Experiments in all scientific fields conceal some aspects of reality while revealing others. This constraint is not unique to those interested in children, or to psychologists. But it poses special issues when one is trying to understand the minds of the creatures we once were. That is, understanding children is different from understanding rocks, nonhuman primates, or adults. I believe that we need to go in both directions: imagine the child implied by various studies, and see how that child matches up to the one we think we encounter in everyday life and, equally important, imagine the child we encounter in everyday life, and try and figure out what kinds of theories might account for what we see.

Because of Piaget and his descendants, I know that during the early years children have a great drive toward making sense of the world. They avidly detect patterns, seek and construct order, and constantly develop strategies to solve the problems they encounter in everyday life—and much of this happens while children are at play. What changes in the first seven or so years of life? The patterns children identify are increasingly abstract and fundamental. The order they construct is increasingly flexible and complex (involving both paradigmatic and narrative orderings). They are more and more likely to integrate fictional with real accounts of experience. The solutions children come up with are increasingly powerful and generalizable (they can apply them to broad ranges of problems and problem types). Their thinking becomes ever more symbolic, and thus abstract.

Children also become increasingly able to think about their own strategies for thinking. Which is why although the four-year-old is likely to remember four, six, or eight items on a list but have no idea how she did it, the eight-year-old can and does monitor her own remembering and think about how to help herself remember (organize information, repeat information, use mnemonics, avoid distractions, and so on). Along the same lines, children are increasingly able to talk about their own feelings and understand the feelings of others.

This brief summary of seventy years of valuable research may seem cursory. But one of the dangers of specialization is that we psychologists get lost in our specific domains of inquiry and forget that there is a larger picture—the child. What do children think and feel, and how does the world look to them? What changes take place in the inner life during these all important early years? In what ways might our understanding of rational aspects of the child's mind be richer and more apt if we could also look more closely and carefully at the less rational processes with which they are intertwined?

Much of the research that has been done since Piaget is ingenious, convincing, and impressive. But when one tries to pull it all together, the picture it gives of young children's minds doesn't resemble enough any child that one might encounter in real life. Some studies focus on thinking, and often try to "take out" the emotion, or control it. Other studies focus on emotion, but rarely examine the child's feelings in the context of complex cognitive activity. Somehow the images of wild child and scientist, implicit in much research as well as in everyday educational and child-rearing practices, have led us to think that the child must be one or the other, and that any given set of phenomena (like, say, problem solving or forming a relationship) must be guided by one strand or the other (feeling or thought). We need a working image of the child that focuses instead on the ways in which feeling and thought, pretense and reality, are intertwined, if not fused, in actual development.

Finally, although many studies use play as a window onto mental development, we still don't know much about what children think and feel as they play. We have only just begun to find ways to describe and understand the psychological chemistry of feeling and thought in young children. Recently I was sitting at a restaurant with a colleague who is an accomplished developmental psychologist and our families. Right next to us was a mother holding her eight-month-old son. The little boy, Ethan, began to stare at my colleague's wife, who gazed back, enchanted, and began talking to Ethan. I said, "Oh boy. Look how excited he is to look at you and see you look back. He looks suffused with feeling." Almost simultaneously my colleague said, "Look. He's clasping his hands together just as you are. He's imitated your gesture." It should be no surprise that we were both probably right. Add to this the pervasive importance of play as both an activity and an orientation in childhood, and one begins to see what a new view of young children must encompass. The challenge for researchers is to describe and investigate the ways in which affectively charged, unconstrained, and imaginative processes are inextricably intertwined with the child's rational processes. What might such a multidimensional view encompass?

3 Spheres of Reality in Childhood

As neuroscientist Susan Greenfield once wrote, "Locked away in our brains is an absolute and inviolate individuality, a personal inner privacy of cascades of thoughts and feelings to which no one else has automatic access."[1] If the adult mind contains this kind of mystery, how much more tantalizingly inaccessible is the mind of the young child? Though each of us has experienced childhood, we find it difficult, if not impossible, to recall what life felt like before we were twelve. Certainly we have no way of thinking back to how we learned things, how we organized knowledge, what distinctions we made, or what kinds of strategies we used to solve mental problems. Moreover, few psychologists these days trust introspection as a means of gaining knowledge about the inner workings of the mind, even among adults.

One way to deal with the mystery of the child's inner mental life is to avoid knowing about it. One might focus instead on what can be pinned down: ages at which various abilities emerge, conditions under which skills can be enhanced or acquired sooner, and influences on various aspects of the child's developing self. But too often this leads us to know more and more about ever narrower issues related to children. If we are to understand the workings of children's minds —how they construe events and what kinds of thoughts and feelings are salient to them in various situations—we will need to find a way to ask about their rich and often messy inner lives.

Implicit in Greenfield's idea of a cascade of thoughts and feelings is the notion that movement and change are integral to the inner mind. With young children, this flux is perhaps more vivid and visible than it is for most adults—it may in fact distinguish the thinking of children between the ages of two and six from that of babies and adults.

As I began this book, a colleague asked me what metaphor I would propose instead of wild child or scientist to describe young children. He suggested explorer; I considered artist. But replacing those old metaphors with a new one misses the point. We can no more capture children's minds with a single metaphor than we could capture the essence of adulthood with one phrase or image. Children are too multifaceted, and vary too much across contexts, to be accurately conveyed through a single image. The urge, unconscious or deliberate, to characterize children with a single metaphor comes from our sense, or hope, that children are simpler than adults, or that they are the same as adults, only less so. Ironically, this "same but less so" view, while prevalent among psychologists, educators, and parents, violates one of Piaget's most profound insights. Though not often amplified by his followers, one of his major themes was that children are qualitatively different from adults. It is not simply that they know less, or have fewer inhibitions, but that the way they think about and encounter the world is unique to their stage of development.

In this chapter, then, I will propose a somewhat different way of characterizing the young child. There is a way to view children that encompasses their scientific as well as wild sides, and in doing so we can describe what is uniquely childlike about children. Such a view should render our understanding of specific processes and abilities (such as numerical reasoning, or thoughts about other people's thoughts) more accurate. I take as a crucial starting point the premise that certain activities and orientations pervade childhood and seem, if not unique, then at least distinctive to early childhood, and that these activities and orientations probably hold the richest information about children's inner lives. Early in life, play seeps into almost every aspect of a child's experience, and is one of the most important and distinct characteristics of early childhood, offering us vital clues about how children both construe the world and navigate the boundaries that give shape to their experience.

THE VITAL CLUE: PLAY

The first thing to note about play will seem obvious to most developmental psychologists and parents: when they have the choice to do so, young children in our culture spend a great deal of time playing. I have yet to come across a culture in which children do not play, though the kinds and amount of play, as well as parental attitudes toward play, vary among individuals, families, and cultures. While psychologists have offered a range of definitions of play, most agree that it involves activity that is in some way intrinsically meaningful to the player, and is marked, at one level or another, as "not for real." Most of us think of play in terms of certain kinds of activity (dress-up, tag, building with blocks, and so on), but it is more fruitful to think of play as a stance one takes toward the activity. Those who know three-year-olds, for example, know that they can be engaged in the most practical real-world activity—unloading groceries, eating cereal, or waiting on line with a parent, and in the blink of an eye have found a way to make the groceries into growling animals, turn the cereal-eating into a game of who can stuff more in quicker, and play peek-a-boo with an adult farther ahead in line. In other words, play may involve activities as self-evident as building with blocks, enacting roles, or transforming everyday objects into weapons and vehicles. But we know that children are playing when they signal, with words, actions, or their nonverbal responses, that their activity is "not real," or "as if." Children are at play when their actions are intrinsically meaningful, and not in the service of some other goal. For instance, imagine a three-year-old boy stacking cards because his father has asked him to put away his toys. The goal of cleaning up makes the activity of stacking a kind of work. But when that child becomes absorbed by the way the cards balance on top of one another, then the goal of cleaning up is pushed aside in favor of the experience of stacking—and he will go on stacking whether the room is cleaned up or not. The child has adopted a playful orientation, which changes the activity in a significant way.

In the past, developmental researchers have focused on play in two ways. Many have used play as a window onto children, using it as a means to study other processes—for instance, children's language, their social relationships, the development of gender, and their ability to solve various kinds of cognitive problems. In these examples, an experimenter elicits some kind of play to better see the behavior being studied; for instance, children sorting blocks will show what kinds of concepts they are able to use for sorting tasks. Other researchers, though far fewer, have been interested in play itself: what kinds of things children play, how play changes as children develop, individual differences in play style, and cultural differences in the importance and role of play for children.[2] Both approaches provide important and valuable information. But both are also problematic, because they overlook a key feature of children's play—it permeates everyday life, influencing every mental process it accompanies. Play that is defined and initiated by the experimenter is quite unlike the play that children regularly initiate and participate in, nor is it simply an activity that can be described like other activities such as household chores, talk, or sibling care. Play is not a unified activity that happens only at a certain time of day, nor can one separate play from the other tasks around which it is wound, such as problem solving or making friends. Playfulness is an orientation toward reality, and thus is central to most of a child's experience. A playful stance can become salient whether a child is sitting on the toilet, filling out a worksheet, or talking to an adult.

What stands out when one watches young children in their natural settings is that the playful orientation seems to come and go. Not only do children move in and out of a "this is play" frame, but in fact they move in and out of a multitude of frames—some pretend, others more oriented toward practical matters. Let me illustrate this idea with two examples.

Recently I walked into the three- and four-year-old room at a nearby day care center. Because I usually go there with the mindset of a psychologist, I often watch with a certain theoretical framework in mind, or a set of empirical questions. This particular morning I was thinking about whether children and adults differ in the distinctions they make between real and not real, and whether the difference is gradual or involves a qualitative leap. Then I sat down and began watching the three- and four-year-olds.

Two little boys, one three-and-a-half years old, the other just over four years old, were standing on opposite sides of a sand table. They were manipulating small figures and blocks in the sand.

The first boy said, in an excited and somewhat awestruck voice, "Magic. Crocodiles." He paused. The second little boy said, "Shovels are not magic." The first little boy said, "You ruined my trick." There was a brief pause, while they both continued to stand at the sand table, and as they chatted with the teacher, who was sitting nearby and talking to them very quietly about turf rights within the sandbox. The first boy then began again, "Magic!" Each time he tried to draw the other child into a discussion of magic, or an appreciation of the magic of crocodiles, the second little boy responded by discussing the politics of turf—who can play with what toy, who can pretend what, and so on.

Nearby, two little girls were playing in the dress-up corner. They were standing side by side, facing a wall, with their backs to me. Each was speaking on a wall phone, for which there was no cord. Each was clearly talking to a husband: "Yes honey, I'll be home later." One little girl had her hand on her hip. They hung up the phones and drifted over to the center of the dress-up corner, where they had made a square out of blocks. One of the girls put her stuffed cat inside the block structure. She looked over at the teacher, and with an almost incomprehensible speech impediment said, "I making a pen for my dat. It's my cat. I making a pen." The teacher replied, "You're making a pen? And why is that?" The child looked at her as if she has missed the obvious: "So she won't get out!"

Then she told the teacher that her cat's name was Glenda. The other little girl said that her baby too was called Glenda. She continued by informing the teacher that Glenda was a nice witch. The teacher responded, "Yes, Glenda is a good witch. I like Glenda; she wears sparkly clothes." This prompts the first child to clarify for the teacher, "But MY Glenda doesn't, isn't—cats don't wear clothes."

Sitting in the corner of a day care center, an observer is struck immediately by how brimming with mental activity the place is. Children are busily negotiating property rights (who will play where), social arrangements (who can play with whom), and rules (what is allowed by other children and grown-ups). But perhaps subtler and even more fascinating, children are energetically defining their own activity and exploring the possibilities within these domains. For instance, the two little boys have somewhat different ideas of what can be done at the sand table, and what roles pretense, magic, and transformation have there. Using both words and gestures, they each define the activity for themselves and one another. Transitions are often subtle and happen quickly. At one point a child may be pretending a small block is a crocodile and the next minute he may be interested in the sand itself and what he can make with it. At this point, the block may serve simply as a block or barrier. Such transformations (redesignating spaces, objects, and one's own role) are happening all over the room. Sometimes these acts of transformation happen seamlessly. But just as often a child will comment on the transformation or show in some way that she is interested or worried about how actions and objects should be interpreted—by herself and others.

In both of these examples we hear children discussing the status of objects. In the second account, however, the little girl confronts a gap, a moment when the teacher seems not to understand that she is speaking from within a play realm (when she explains that the pen is there to keep the cat from getting out). Further, when she explains to the teacher that her Glenda is not the same as her friend's Glenda because a cat can't wear clothes, she is straddling two levels of reality and trying to put this into words. On the one hand, she is accepting the idea that one or both of the toys can be Glenda, and on the other hand, she is drawing the line at the notion that her Glenda, which is a toy cat, could wear clothes.

For those of us interested in pretend play, it has been common to think the child's world was divided into pretend/nonpretend (play/work, imaginary/real). This is too simplistic, suggesting an overly stable, firm line between types of experience. The child's world is probably more multifaceted than that, and less fixed. Children more likely experience their world as a configuration of sometimes overlapping spheres—domains of experience that are defined not only by what the child is doing, but also by how she approaches the activity and interprets the experience of doing that activity. Children's spheres of experience are not stable or firm, but rather are created and negotiated by children as they act in the world. What then, are these spheres, and how do children go about using them?

Spheres of Experience

Heinz Werner was one of the first and only developmental theorists to focus on tracing the changing relationships between rational and irrational thinking during childhood.[3] This interest grew in part out of his emphasis on the importance of investigating children's experience of themselves and the world, rather than their capacities. As Margery Franklin has explained in her discussion of Werner's theory, "A person's experience does not mirror external reality as physically defined, but reflects the shaping forces of needs, interests, expectations, and cognitive structurings . . . how human beings act within and upon their surrounds, and in relation to others, issues from their subjective experiential structurings of their surrounds."[4] In other words, Werner's interest in experience led to a developmental theory that attempted to account not only for observable changes in children's performance, but also for the relationship between such performances and their motivations, feelings, and thoughts about the world in which they were functioning.

Werner argued that babies and young children initially experience the world globally—that is, as one fused experience in which, for example, the domains of self and other, symbol and referent, and reality and fantasy are merged. Development entails, in his view, an increasing differentiation between domains, with, for instance, the baby beginning to realize that he is separate from his mother, that words and the things he names are not the same, and that the realm of make-believe is separate from that of practical, everyday reality. As these domains become differentiated, they also become more distinct. Specifically, as children become aware of the difference between what is real and what is imagined, what is playful and what is pragmatic, the boundaries between these types of experience become firmer.[5] As the opening examples of the boys at the sand table and the girls with the toy cats convey, one of the most interesting aspects of children's behavior is the way in which they seem to move back and forth between these spheres. Children often seem as interested in the boundaries of such spheres, and in crossing those boundaries, as they are in whatever goes on within the sphere.

By the time children can use symbols to transform reality in stories or in gesture, they have become interested in moving back and forth between spheres. Visualize, for instance, a child sponging a table after snack time, who begins to make patterns of water on the table, and then, after a few moments, uses the sponge to enact an airplane flying over the table, complete with engine noises. Though Werner argued that the young child makes little distinction between fantasy and reality, he was probably putting it too strongly. We know that most three-year-olds pretending that a stuffed dog is their pet would be shocked—and probably horrified—if the dog suddenly started barking and moving. But Werner was pointing us in the right direction by emphasizing the importance of the child's orientation toward experience. A four-year-old child's approach to playing "baby puppy" is different in quality and intensity from the way a nine-year-old might engage in such play. That is, it is not simply the case that the four-year-old and the nine-year-old might give different answers to questions about the ontological status of the dog, but that they experience "pretend" differently. This experiential difference is extremely important and cannot be detected simply in children's ability to explain what is going on.

Children are usually riveted by what happens within their pretend frame. But they often seem equally interested in creating the frame and then crossing it, inviting others into it, breaking it up, or reshaping it. One visible sign of young children's interest in their own spheres of experience can be found in the way they talk about pretending and not pretending. Conversations like the one in which the two boys discuss whether shovels can be magic illustrate this point. It may be surprising for the casual observer to realize that children talk about pretending as much as they actually pretend, and that this talk is in fact an integral part of the experience.

Creating and Crossing Boundaries

In recent years there has been renewed interest in the kinds of thinking that children use when they are pretending. Paul Harris has argued that children's play often contains sequences and scenarios that use the same logic as everyday life.[6] Play dialogues and play gestures don't have their own set of rules or cognitive processes, as some had previously argued. Instead, it is the frame—the fictive world itself—that differentiates play from not play, real from not real. Angeline Lillard has described this same notion in a particularly vivid fashion. She likens the alternate world of pretend to the philosopher's "Twin Earth," an imagined planet in which everything is pretty much as it is in the "real world." By adopting this perspective, the philosopher can speculate on what might happen in the real world "if only."[7] If, in fact, children cross a boundary to function in a "twin Earth" pretend sphere, how and when do they learn to make that crossing? To answer this question, Lillard has begun to examine the ways in which mothers signal to their toddlers that they are pretending. In video clips one can see mothers using a special voice, and gesturing in an exaggerated way, when they want their child to know they are pretending something—for instance, to drink tea out of a toy tea cup.

When a child pretends, much of what happens within their pretense parallels, if not mimics, the thoughts, activities, and content of everyday, nonpretend life. But when it is framed by a pretend orientation, the experience is very different for the child. It was the anthropologist Gregory Bateson who first described the power of a play frame, in his descriptions of young apes who play fight. He pointed out that the primates engage in the very actions (biting, hitting, and so on) that would lead to injury, or death, under other circumstances. But the primates are able to communicate to themselves and one another the message "this is play," so that all the actions carried out within that frame are not taken literally.[8] The same can be said for the American game of football. If a man rushed up and jumped on another man in the street, it could lead to a horrible fight, perhaps injury or death, and certainly arrest. But if both men know they are "playing football," the same actions that might lead to a fight, lead instead to a game. Researchers refer to actions that seem real, but are not, as being in the "as if" mode. When a child goes through all the motions of sitting down and drinking tea, the only thing that marks it as play is the "as if" orientation of the players. All the actions within such a mode are nearly identical to the actions used in a real episode of drinking tea. In the past, most researchers have assumed that there were two domains: everyday life, to be taken literally, and pretend activity, the "as if" domain. But there is more than one way to pretend, and possibly more than one pretend sphere. Consider the following episode. Three children are playing house. One picks up a phone, which was clearly once a real phone, though not plugged in anymore, and passes it to another boy. "It's your Mom." The other boy takes the phone and says, "Oh, hi Dad." He then hands a toy banana to a third child, and says, "This can be your phone. You're the dad."

These children are not confused about whether their moms and dads are really on the phone, or whether those are real phones. Their use of objects (including both a nonfunctioning phone and a banana) as if they were phones is what matters. But within the domain designated as play, the "as if" world, they are enacting a "what is" scenario—real kinds of conversations between moms and dads and their children. Pretending realistically is not only prevalent in early childhood, but also extremely important, providing children with opportunities to understand and master aspects of everyday life—rehearsing scripts, consolidating knowledge of social reality, assimilating confusing or charged events, and so on. But children also use the pretense frame to explore more far-fetched possibilities. In the following example, for instance, there is much greater interest in nonrealistic pretense.

Two little boys are playing in the day care center with some small cars, planes, and rockets. One of the boys, earlier interested in magic crocodiles at the sandbox, is now manipulating a small toy rocket. He zooms one through the air, saying to the other little boy, "Magic. Watch. 3-2-1, Blast off! (Makes a series of blasting noises with his mouth.) Magic, huh?" Then he walks over to me holding the rocket and says, "This rocket flies because it has a blaster." This sentence is a perfect example of the dual status of his play. The rocket is a toy, but at that moment it can fly and blast. Yet his explanation of why the rocket flies is perfectly reasonable. If he were a guide at NASA showing me around, he might utter exactly the same words. Perhaps more interesting is the fact that the little boy thinks he has to account for why the rocket can fly. That means that a play frame or boundary can make the toy possess real attributes (blasting and flying). But the flying rocket still requires real-life explanations.

The child draws an "as if" line around the rocket. This is exactly what Harris means when he says that the child uses regular real-world logic and thinking, but within a fictive world. If Harris and Lillard are correct, then some of the time what young children do and think within a play frame is only different from more real-life activity because of the boundary around it. This underscores the power of such frames in shaping real-life experience and guiding its interpretation.

From What Is to What If

The play frame also allows children to draw on forms of thinking and logic that are not related to the real world. Some of the time children enter an "as if" world in order to explore "what if" scenarios. When children construct play scenarios in which impossible things happen, or where they use magic to explain surprising events, they are exploring the sphere of "what if." In the following example, a three-year-old girl is not only pretending—that is, she not only takes an "as if" stance toward everyday experience; she also creates a kind of experience that she cannot have had or seen in real life. She has created a sphere of "what if."

> Wanna go, wanna fly, wanna fly together? Here my wings. Here these can be your wings. C'mon in, sky. Ok. Now you warn the baby animals that rain is coming. "We're coming babies. Don't worry. We're coming. We'll save you."

This kind of play, which so clearly hangs on a narrative framework, entails a kind of speculative thinking and rearranging of the experienced world that "what is play" does not contain.

The lines around these spheres need to be frequently restated and reconsidered by the young players. The same two girls who were playing with their babies and their cat moved the cat and one baby to a new area, where they set about building the cat a new cage. One little girl held a doll and said first to herself, and then to me, "That's my baby." Then she paused, pointed to the stuffed cat, and said, "That kitten is real." It is hard to know what this statement does for the little girl, or what it means to her. Perhaps she is caught for a moment—uncertain of the play boundary, even confused by her own statement that the doll is her baby. She may need to fortify or reestablish the status of her toys as real. The underlying message of her statement might be, "Let's just remember that I am pretending that these toys are real, and that they stand for a real baby and a real cat." It is also possible that at that moment she has become aware that I am watching, and knows enough about the interpersonal dynamic of establishing play frames to realize that I may not understand that she is playing. She may think that I need to be told the status of the toys. An elegantly designed study might establish which of these interpretations is most accurate—that she is reaffirming the status of her toys for herself, or establishing a joint pretend frame with me. But the truth is probably messier than that. The truth is, she may be talking for herself and for me, as well as expressing her uncertainty about the status of the toy. Playing with the boundary may be part of what is gratifying to her about the activity. In fact, sometimes it is apparent that a child is defining her sphere as "what if" and trying to figure out what makes that sphere different from others. Consider the following example. A three-year-old girl is playing in the bath with two plastic lions representing Simba and Nahla, two characters from the movie *The Lion King*. She is using them to enact a happily-ever-after scenario, repeating versions of "The prince is going to marry the princess and live happily ever after." Her father, who is shaving nearby, tries to join the play by saying, "And what about Pumba? Is he going to get married?" The little girl stops her playing, and with a steely stare at her father says, "In your precious world there is nothing. There is no happily ever after. No talking!" and returns to playing with the two plastic tigers. She has drawn a circle around her imaginary play, and clearly thinks that happily ever after belongs within that circle, a circle that excludes her father and his world.

Sometimes one need only watch a child's gestures to see her switch frames. I once saw a little girl holding a doll in an amazingly realistic fashion, just as a competent relaxed mother or older sister might hold a baby, with a hand under the baby's bottom and one at her back. She then placed the baby in a little toy high chair, quite careful to make the baby comfortable and stable. One might speculate that the baby who needed its back supported is a lot younger than the baby who can sit in a high chair, but no matter—the next moment is much more dramatic. At this point the little girl turns her attention toward another part of the dress-up area, and as she does so the doll tips over, hanging by its foot on the footrest of the high chair. Interested now by the clothes in another part of the doll corner, the little girl pays no attention to the dangling baby, though she can plainly see what has happened. Clearly the play designation "this is real" has been suspended.

Significantly, the child's day is not entirely devoted to what adults recognize as pretend play. Many hours are filled with straightforward transactions. These will vary from one community to another.[9] In my community, for instance, these might include such important daily chores as saying goodbye to Daddy at day care, getting dressed and undressed, cleaning up the blocks, eating lunch, and so forth. In addition, at least for many children, there are hours of play that involve less pretense and more building, patterning, and moving around. For instance, walk into a good day care center at the beginning of the day, and two children will be playing daddy in the dress-up corner, two or three others will be putting together a jigsaw puzzle, one child will be aimlessly wandering around humming a little tune and vaguely touching various items, and another child will be pretending to read a book to herself in the book corner.

In each case, whether pretense is salient or not, it may well be only a part of the child's orientation toward the task. In one example of this, a little boy, four years old, was putting together some Legos to create some kind of vehicle with a figure at the helm. A second boy wandered over and stood watching for a moment. "Remember, remember when we were playing Luke Skywalker before? Remember that? Wanna play that game again?" The little boy nodded, and the second boy settled down to build his own Lego contraption. What is interesting here is that building (what psychologist Dennie Wolf calls modeling—focusing on the physical properties of objects and their interrelationships) is probably the most important part of what they each are doing.[10] And yet at least for one of the children, putting it in the context of an imaginary framework (playing Luke Skywalker) adds something important to the experience. Moment by moment, choosing colors, figuring out how to make them fit, or adding new pieces is what is most absorbing and demanding. A little while later, the same boy who wanted to make it a Luke Skywalker game pointed his creation at the first boy and said, "I'm shooting you. This is a shooting and fighting game." The second boy shook his head. "No you can't. No fighting, Laurie said. No shooting." The first boy continued pointing the toy and making little shooting noises, saying, "Well, I am." A minute later they are each distracted by goings-on in the room. And yet about five minutes later the small shooter has launched himself at the first boy, and they get into something of a scuffle.

The point here is not that one child is violent and the other is not. Instead this sequence of behavior illustrates two aspects of childhood: first, children's behavior rarely fits into one category. The same activity may serve several functions simultaneously, or one after another in rapid succession. Second, a common theme, whether cognitive or emotional, may follow a child through a series of interactions that appear quite distinct. Pretend play is an excellent vehicle for allowing children to explore a theme again and again. The theme may have emotional pull for the child, or may simply represent a topic, event, or puzzle that interests him intellectually.

Emotion as Fuel for Play

Not all play contains potent emotional material, and psychologists still disagree about the value of interpreting children's play for underlying affective content. But it is hard, as well as counterproductive, to ignore the emotional content that children are drawn to when playing because such content offers yet another example of the ways in which the child's world is usually multilayered. In a paper outlining the dramatic play of one little two-year-old, the clinician Elsa First describes a little girl, Jane, who introduces a favorite game in which she is leaving someone and the person must cry. For instance, on one occasion while playing with her mother the little girl says, "I'm going. You be alone. You cry." The little girl plays variations of this again and again with her father, her mother, and her babysitter.[11] Certainly the little girl is exploring the structure and mechanics of dramatic play. She assigns roles, directs action, and articulates a sequence that includes a high point. But it seems misguided to ignore her choice of topics, given what we know about the importance of attachment to two-year-olds. She certainly seems to be exploring a potent emotional theme: leaving and being left. What we still don't know is how the affective potency of a theme relates to the cognitive pull of the process for young children. It is at least plausible, from what we already know, that children exploit their budding cognitive skills in the service of potent emotional themes. To weed out the emotional force of children's activity from its cognitive structure is difficult at best, and bad science at worst. Why are young children compelled to play, make up stories, or draw? Clearly one reason is that the imagined worlds they construct in play provide them with vital opportunities for developing and practicing important cognitive tools. But the charged themes that often pervade children's play suggest that emotions are an equally important force. We have some evidence of this from recent research on the emotional content of young children's stories. Robert Emde and his colleagues have developed an impressive research program designed to identify the emotions of young children. They provide three-year-old children with story beginnings, called "story stems," and ask them to complete the story. Their analyses of the resulting narratives identify a wide range of children's feelings and give a glimpse of what Emde calls the "inner worlds" of the young child.[12]

It is typical rather than unusual for a child to suggest a theme such as "I leave and you cry" for her dramatic play. Other typical scenarios involve some catastrophe a child has heard a great deal about (a blackout, a flood, a car accident), or even less dramatic events that loom large in the life of a young child (the birth of a sibling, a family trip, or the death of a pet). It must be noted that the interaction can work in the opposite way as well. Many clinicians have observed that too much anxiety can prevent a child from playing.[13] But it is not only that children use play as a way of rehearsing or reenacting potent emotional material. It is also the case that play can create or trigger emotions.

Harris has provided evidence for this idea. When he and his colleagues read sad stories to children, they found that the children's mood was markedly more somber afterward than it had been before. They could not attribute this to any confusion between what is real and what is imagined, since in a separate set of studies children far younger had shown a clear ability to tell the difference between an imaginary friend and a real friend, a made-up story and what had really happened, or a toy animal and its real counterpart. In other words, children's moods are influenced by fictive material.[14]

Play and emotion obviously have a complex and dynamic way of interacting in the life of the young child. This interaction exemplifies the idea that what a child experiences within one sphere may color what she experiences within another sphere. A child who has played something that aroused angry feelings may well feel angry while later picking up her toys, or attending to a baby sibling. A child who had an upsetting fall at day care may play "falling down" at home for days afterward. Play and nonplay spheres influence one another throughout the child's day, and within the child's mind.

FROM PLAY TO STORYTELLING

Pretend play is not the only way that children symbolize and express complex inner meanings. Storytelling is one of the most prevalent ways young children mold, communicate, and sometimes reflect on their own complex inner thoughts and feelings. Like pretend play, many stories told by children between the ages of two and around seven offer a wonderful window onto the ways in which strong feeling and newly emerging forms of thought come together. Examining children's stories provides one excellent way to begin to tease apart the spheres of experience that are central to young children.

I am not the first to propose that stories give children the means to make fundamental distinctions in their organization of reality. In describing the ways in which narratives guide people's formulation of experience, Jerome Bruner and Joan Lucariello argued that toddlers use stories to sort out the canonical from the noncanonical; the usual from the unusual. For instance, in their now classic analysis of a toddler who talked herself to sleep each night in her crib, Bruner and Lucariello describe how Emily would often go over the day, talking about what "usually" happens, what might happen, and something special, exciting, or worrisome that had happened. Bruner and Lucariello argued that, by definition, narratives distinguish canonical from noncanonical. In this way, they suggest, the narrative form drives our construction of experience.[15]

While play is the main activity of three- and four-year-olds in our culture, it recedes during the first eight years of life, until its earliest form all but disappears. Storytelling, however, in all its manifestations, not only appears early in life, but also remains a central way that people make sense of their world and communicate with others.

The Many Spheres within Stories

Some stories fit our models of narrative development, but many of the most interesting ones do not. We don't yet really understand how it is that children use narrative as a means of construing their worlds. Many of the stories children spontaneously tell or write look very little like the ones investigated in good experiments. They are often enigmatic, confusing, idiosyncratic, and whimsical. Often young children's narratives and narrative fragments do not fit logical models—even the models created to capture the thinking of young children. Nevertheless, children's stories, enacted, spoken, and written, are brimming with meaning. They can tell us a lot about not only what a child is thinking, but also how he is thinking. Our task is to find some general principles that describe or explain narratives, or tell us what narratives reveal about a child's mind, without losing sight of their specificity and originality—the meaning that makes narratives so interesting and important to study in the first place.

Over the last twenty years there has been an explosion of information and insight about the ways in which young children become adept storytellers. We know that with age children become more independent as storytellers—more able to tell a complete story without the support and contributions of an adult conversational partner. We know that early on their stories are often only fragments or germs of stories: they may not have a beginning or an end, they may lack a problem or high point, they may not offer resolutions, and they may overlook a commentary that directs the audience's interpretation.

We also know that as children develop, their stories become more "regular," that is, more like the stories of adults in their community. Older children create stories that are less idiosyncratic, revealing, dynamic, and expressive of a specific view of the world, or at least those levels of meaning become harder to dig out of the story. Contrast, for instance, these two stories, both told as "real life" accounts of cats. The first was dictated by a five-year-old:

> This is a cat walking.
> The cat is still walking.
> The cat is walking to the graveyard.
> Pearl is cute and she is beautiful. Meow.
> My cat, Pearl, is walking a lot.
> Pearl is eating.
> Pearl finds her home.
> And this is night time.

This second story was written by a nine-year-old in school:

> Once there was a frog named Herb. He lived on the window sill of the Morris Family. Herb liked to eat flies, but he couldn't always catch enough to fill him up. One day he decided to jump into the kitchen of

> the Morris family and try some human food. So he jumped onto the kitchen table and ate up their cereal. But then the daughter, named Maggie, walked in. Oh no she screamed, a frog . . . But then she saw that he was really cute. She went over and picked him up. After that Herb lived inside and ate his meals with the Morris family.

These examples suggest that as children get older, their stories become more conventional and therefore less crafted by and reflective of the author's inner life. They also support the tendency for researchers and educators to see narrative development as a kind of neat progression toward orderliness, logic, and comprehensibility.[16]

But when children are between the ages of two-and-a-half and five they energetically and enthusiastically, if unconsciously, exploit the potential for using narrative as a way to construe and reconstrue their world. That is, they simultaneously explore their world through narratives and explore narratives themselves. This dynamic and often messy-looking activity has not been captured well in our research. We haven't yet found ways to make sense of these more idiosyncratic stories children tell, though they may ultimately be the most interesting ones to try and understand.

When children tell a story, they create a world. Each story not only describes a cast of characters and a series of events; it also sets forth characteristics that define a particular sphere of reality. Within that world, things happen in a certain way. So, for instance, a child might tell a story in which objects can be people, past events shape future events, or thoughts and feelings are preeminent, with action or events invisible or unimportant. Children use the story form and the act of telling a story to draw a boundary around the events contained in the narrative, in much the same way that children often use words, objects, and actions to create a boundary around their play that lets themselves and others know that the actions are, in Bateson's words, "real and not real at the same time."

The literary scholar Samuel Levin has said that every poem has an invisible first line: "I invite you into a world in which." Levin argues that that implied first line signals to the reader that the metaphors within the poem are to be taken literally. In the world of that particular poem, sadness is literally a cloud, or man is literally a wolf, and so on.[17] I would like to extend that idea here and suggest that when a child begins a story, whether she is telling it to someone else or telling it as an accompaniment to her play, she delineates and announces a world in which the actions and events she names are real. In other words, once she has signaled to herself or another that she has taken an "as if" orientation toward events, the actions and characters she depicts feel, for that moment, real to her. Without such force, stories wouldn't have the kind of psychological power that they clearly have. Each story offers the child a world in which, for instance, objects have personalities, time moves backward and forward, boundaries between domains are permeable, and the relationship between symbols and referents is shifting. The actions and characters in a story are compelling, arouse emotions, and have an effect on both the tellers and the listener. Yet the sentences and descriptions are not actually those actions and characters; instead they are vivid versions of reality safely circumscribed within the narrative frame. Everything said within a narrative boundary is subject to internal rules, rather than external rules—what Bruner meant when he said a narrative is indifferent to facts.[18] This is why some of the time children use real-world logic within their play and narratives, as Harris and Lillard have argued, and at other times draw on nonlogical forms of thinking such as magic. Children construct stories as a way of exploring spheres or provinces of meaning, but they also explore boundaries between spheres or provinces.

Narratives offer an especially powerful vehicle for exploring boundaries between spheres of reality because they carry with them both the meanings and distinctions important to the culture, as well as the potential to rearrange such meanings using narrative techniques. In that sense narratives are a potent tool for thinking because they are simultaneously bound by real-world rules and expectations, and can also violate those rules. A story that bears no reference to our lived experience would be uninteresting and incomprehensible. But one that is no more than a dry record isn't a story. The power of stories lies in their ability to oscillate between spheres. This oscillation is exactly what we see in many narratives created by young children.

A colleague has shared with me that as a young boy he often told himself stories about playing baseball. In these stories he would begin by describing something that he recalled from an actual Little League game in which he had played. At some point the story would begin to change. Fiction would replace remembered events, as he accomplished heroic plays that won the game. He says, "Mostly I told these inside my head. But they were vivid, and I would often repeat the same story several times, sometimes changing certain details. Once in a while I even began saying a certain story out loud to myself. But I don't think I ever told anyone." As his account demonstrates, the line between secret inner stories and shared public stories is a movable one. What can begin as a completely silent story can then become spoken, yet still told only when one is alone. At some other time that same story might find its way into a more public arena. His stories of baseball heroism also moved back and forth between what he recalled from a real incident and what he wished might happen. These types of fluidity reflect the psychological power of children's storytelling. The ways in which children may slide back and forth between what happened and what might have happened is an important aspect of early development.

An equally interesting part of the developmental picture is the way in which children acquire a conscious awareness of such boundaries. A parent once offered me a good example of this in a story about her two daughters, ages four and six. The four-year-old was going on and on, while riding in the car, about the many things that had happened to her in school. The story sounded to the mother's ears as if only some of it was plausible ("They served pizza for lunch, and a huge bear came into the room and grabbed the pizza. . ."). The older daughter ran a quiet steady commentary on her sister's narrative, "True, not true, not true, true." Children use stories (their own and other people's) to differentiate between what they consider to be fact and what they believe to be fiction.

In recent years, psychologists have viewed narrative as the vehicle through which children become socialized. Thus great emphasis has been placed on the ways in which children learn shared habits of mind and interaction through their storytelling. With an increased excitement about what narratives can tell us, and the seeming accessibility of their meanings, has come a gradual shift in focus, from thinking of narratives as a solitary and private activity to considering them a pursuit that is visible, apprehensible.[19] This mirrors the general trend I have described toward thinking of children as increasingly knowable, socialized, and rational.

Constructing a story does many things for a child, just as it does for the storytelling adult. One function of storytelling for the young child is to create a bridge between the self and important others (friends, teachers, and parents). To some extent the developmental paradigm of storytelling has focused on the ways in which children use stories to become members of their communities. Thus a great deal of psychological research has shown how children acquire the storytelling habits and values of the culture, how they become more able to use stories in social interactions, and how those interactions then shape their representations of experience.[20] Another focus of developmental research has been the way in which stories become more logical, more thematically organized, more sequential, and more grammatical as children get older.[21] The implication in much of this research is that stories reflect more general changes in the way children think—from less organized to more organized, from cryptic to explicit, and from idiosyncratic to formal and conventional.

The developmental account of narrative processes has yielded important information about the principled or regular changes that most children exhibit as they age, as well as about the relationship between narrative and other aspects of inter- and intrapersonal processes. This developmental account is convincing, and enlightening, but only to some extent. With all the clarity and systematicness that has emerged from the research, an essential aspect of children's early narratives has been lost. For those of us studying children's narratives from a psychological perspective, it is important to keep in full sight, at all times, the wilderness from which narratives emerge.

The Wild Side of Children's Stories

The unruly nature of children's stories provides vital clues to the child's inner thoughts and fantasies. Stories do conform to social conventions of storytelling, and they do reflect the inner logic of narrative—something that seems to emerge automatically like some other mental shifts, for instance, understanding that the volume of matter doesn't change even when its appearance changes, seeing things and situations from a variety of perspectives, or understanding abstract concepts such as justice. An impressive body of research also shows the ways in which children learn to use the storytelling habits and techniques of their culture. But stories also reflect deeply personal ways of organizing experience. Young children construct stories as a way of wresting meaning from their daily lives.[22] Often their narratives contain evidence of the emotional and cognitive conundrums they are trying to solve, with the form of the narrative hinting at the kinds of solutions the children have devised. The following story, dictated to a teacher by a four-year-old girl, happens to center on the theme of wildness. But more importantly the story is told with many shifts and changes, each reflecting the way in which the child is making sense of experience as she goes along.

> *THE KITTEN THAT WAS WILD*
> There was a kitten that was wild. And it wanted to climb on a tree. The kitten captured and killed a rabbit for breakfast.

The kitten took the rabbit to his sister kitten and a tiger came by.
The kitten was up in a tree and it jumped up higher because it wanted to get a bird. The kitten was going to eat the bird for lunch.
He almost caught the bird, but he only caught a feather and fell into the tree. He climbed on a branch and tried to dig his claws into the branch but couldn't. He fell to the ground and hit his head.
He grew up into a large cat. He could make tracks on trees with his claws. He knocked a coconut down. And he could stand on his hind legs. A hunter came by to kill the cat and he almost caught him but he didn't.
And the cat's tail grew longer. It almost touched the sky.
The horse was crying because his family was lost.
The cat came to help find his family.
Alex and Katie found their family, too.
Alex and Katie were on their floatie in the water. Then they fell off into the water.
The sun was going down and it was reflecting on the water.
They floated to shore.
And they made a campsite.
They walked to the desert.
They kept walking and ended up in the city.
And then they walked to the jungle.
Then Alex got into quicksand. Katie helped Alex get out.
Alex and Katie were sleeping. Then Katie ran away because the tiger came back to them.
Alex ran to the desert to see if Katie was there.
But Katie wasn't there. And he stayed there and stayed there and stayed there . . .
And then he found Katie.
And they were happy forever.

This story contains a range of "problems" the storyteller seems interested in mulling over, such as losing one's family, reuniting with family, wild animals, and the possibility that things will be transformed, for better or for worse. These may not be scary or deep problems, but they seem to interest the storyteller. Creating such a narrative gives her an opportunity to explore, rehearse, and reconfigure troubling, intriguing, and appealing events.[23] The "Kitten That Was Wild" is characteristic of young children's storytelling in that the process of telling appears to be as important to the child as the story itself. In this sense, narrating constitutes a form of play for the storyteller. The story begins as a moment-by-moment account of a kitten trying to eat a bird, and ends as a more epic account of two friends, Alex and Katie, who lose one another and then are reunited. Along the way the kitten becomes a tiger. At times the story reads in a fairly realistic way, and then, abruptly, becomes fantastical. The narrator plays with language, each sentence emerging from the one before, with little if any obvious governing thematic or dramatic principle. The experience of creating scenes and images with words is as satisfying to the young child as making a house with blocks, or enacting a fight between two dolls. Young children's stories, spoken and written, often seem as if they represent the convergence of two kinds of thinking, introduced by Sigmund Freud as primary and secondary process thinking. Primary process refers here to unconscious thinking that is unhampered by rules of everyday logic, drawing instead on a wide range of symbolic processes and forms. Freud considered primary process thinking to be typical of dreaming. Secondary process thinking is the more logical, rule-governed, and conventionally organized thought processes usually employed in waking, task-oriented daily life. Those who still use Freud's framework tend to think of primary process thinking as being id governed while secondary process thinking is ego governed.[24] But even if one rejects the original Freudian construction, it is not hard to see that the kinds of rules we use to formulate and express our experiences and thoughts vary across contexts. Contrast, for instance, the way one thinks while constructing a scientific argument and the way one thinks while fantasizing about something very scary. Children's stories often seem to go back and forth between these two types of thinking. It can be hard to distinguish developmentally immature forms of organization (preconceptual ways of grouping things, for instance) from idiosyncratic ways of structuring experiences that simply express the closeness between the two kinds of thinking (primary and secondary process) in young children.

One of the reasons that narratives provide such a rich window onto the many spheres of childhood is that they allow for and express a multitude of boundaries. For instance, narratives may form a psychological curtain between what is wild and private and what is orderly and public. When children tell stories, they exploit narrative devices to both create and explore the boundary between the two. The young storyteller can actively negotiate the distinctions between what is revealed and what is concealed, between following the conventions of one's culture and breaking those conventions. For instance, a four-year-old came home from preschool one day, and her mother asked her how the day went. The little girl answered readily, "It was fun. I don't like Mrs. Poulos. She's mean. She won't let us talk during snack . . . and then we got so mad at her that all the kids tied her up with rope and left her sitting in the middle of the room." In this narrative the child has glided from reality to fantasy, from what was to what she wished had been. The narrative allows her to connect and compare the two types of reality. And it allows internal experience to become external landscape. Her fantasy of revenge on a feared authority becomes an actual scene with actors, props, and gestures.

Slightly older children also use stories to sort out the seen from the hidden. Their concern with these boundaries is evident not only in their stories, but also in what they say about stories. The parent of a six-year-old boy named Riley, for example, reported that Riley heard an extremely scary ghost story from his much older brother. That night Riley was afraid to go to sleep. Lying worriedly next to his mother, he kept saying, "If I go to sleep I might have a nightmare about it and in the middle of the dream I can't tell that it's not real." Riley has to figure out what he already has a glimmer of: that stories you hear can become internalized and reappear as dreams, and that because dreams feel as if they are actually happening, they are even scarier than a story. One of the benefits of spoken, conscious narratives is that they provide us with the means of putting a fence around scary material. When you tell a story, there are all kinds of soothing indications that it is a story, not actual life. For the young storyteller, this is not only a characteristic of stories, but also a focal point of the storytelling process.

When adult authors use narratives to create boundaries, it usually seems deliberate. Authors such as Philip Roth and Jamaica Kinkaid use autobiography as a screen or curtain that confuses the reader further about what is fact and what is fiction in their writing.[25] But herein lies an important developmental difference. The child uses narrative devices and the narrative form itself to create these spheres of reality for herself as much as for a listener. Through her symbolic action, she creates spheres on which she can reflect. She can explore the boundaries of those spheres, and vary what she reveals and conceals. When the adult author dissembles and plays with boundaries, he does so for an audience.

In the following story, a nine-year-old girl named Ella does a masterful job of both concealing and revealing. Philip Roth could not improve on Ella's artful shift between what is real and what is imagined, and between the types of reality she chooses to express. She simultaneously exposes her inner thoughts and keeps them shrouded.

> I am Ella from Viet Nam. I am in the war. The Americans are attacking us Vietnamese people. I am spying on my sister who is from the U.S. She is in the army too. Sergeant Knuckles is sending me in. Oh I have two Americans on my tail. Good I killed them. Here is the medical doctor taking care of some of our hurt people. It is very dangerous. I just got a foot away from my sister who is known as one of the best fighters in America she is also my evilest sister. I am so glad to be in my tent once again. And to be writing my Mom and Dad a letter.

Just so you know my sister would never write a letter to Mom and Dad only I would. Except she would if it was mean.

Dear Mom and Dad,
I miss you very much. And I know that you worry about me but there is nothing to worry about because with Sergeant Knuckle by my side I will never even have to worry. I love you.
Signed,
Ella

There goes a gun shot. I better track down my sister. Wake up Knuckles, wake up. But he wasn't there, he left a note saying he was by the pond so I ran over there as fast as I could. And there he was laying down dead. Oh no he couldn't be dead. But he was. It is the army so I have to leave him and track down my sister. O.K. back to my journey. I hear my sister, I will find her. But first write a letter to my Mom and Dad.

Dear Mom and Dad,
Sergeant Knuckles died but don't worry, I'll be fine.
I love you.
Love,
Ella

I am tracking my sister down there she is. I am Justine, my sister is Ella and I just shot her now she is dead.

Dear Mom and Dad,
I just killed Ella so too bad. I know when you get this letter you will cry your sorry little butts off but too bad. I hate you.
From Justine.

In this story the author clearly combines fact and fiction. She does have a sister named Justine. She has never been to Vietnam. She has dramatized her view of the family competition for parental love, as all good storytellers do. She is American but chooses to write this from the point of view of a Vietnamese. I have argued elsewhere that children invent and adopt narrative devices (such as perspective, live-action narration, switches in tense, and epistolary communication) in order to convey meaning. Thus when the meaning is rich and potent, the invention and borrowing of literary devices are most active. Here these devices allow the storyteller to come out from behind the curtain, and then slip back behind it, within the space of only two sentences.

One reason the curtain is so visible in Ella's story is that her material is loaded with personal meaning and affect. Bruner has argued that narratives serve as a cooling vessel for children, allowing them to gain first symbolic, and then emotional and cognitive, distance from the experiences they recount. When powerful feelings like rivalry, love, or sexual curiosity take shape in a story, the words and narrative form both embody and contain the feelings, thus giving the narrator distance from her own affect. Where Ella might have had inchoate feeling, she now has constructed a sphere of reality that she can move in and out of. But as author she also has some authority over what is made explicit and what is not. In recent years several psychologists have noted that the silences and omissions in narratives are as important as what is said. Often provocative clues about a child's thoughts or experiences are followed not by amplification but by silence or a complete switch in topics. In other words, the child has pulled the narrative curtain, obscuring her material. She can use stories to both reveal and then conceal.

Ella's story is a vivid example of the kind of emotionally hot material children are most drawn to using in their stories. In this way they are not so different from adults. The difference may lie in what constitutes hot for the young child. In his essay "The Interested Party" from his collection *The Beast in the Nursery*, psychoanalyst Adam Phillips argues that Freud thought curiosity is the natural avenue of sublimation when children's sexual appetite and interest are forced underground.[26] Phillips claims that this explains why society, in the guise, say, of school, ends up discouraging and quelling curiosity, because those who work in and preside over such institutions unconsciously know that curiosity is as dangerous as sex. Phillips also argues that stories provide children with a perfect vehicle for exploring sex, satisfying their curiosity, and seeking pleasure.

The stories themselves are not always about pleasure. But the story form allows children to peek, flirt, imagine, encounter danger, and concretize wishes. Phillips might argue that children's narratives, like their play, often revolve around the body. But I believe that stories represent a first symbolic embodiment of the physical and the sensuous. Telling the story is itself a pleasurable activity. The story may or may not be about the body, but the process of creating events through words and sentences teeters on the boundary between the mental and the physical, between thought and action.

Five Contrasting Themes in Children's Stories

There are certain contrasts or tensions that seem to be particularly salient in young children's stories. So far I have suggested two kinds of boundaries that children create and explore in their play and narratives: the boundary between "what if" and "what is," and the boundary between public and private. But children also create and explore other distinctions as they construe the world around them. Here I identify five different themes that children often integrate into their storytelling as a way of thinking about contrasting possibilities in real-life experience.

One seemingly simple but important detail of my approach is that I look at each story as something that unfolds in real time. A story is a timeless text, but for the child it is a process with a beginning and an end. What a child does in the beginning of a story may be different from what he says or how he says it in the middle of the story. The psychological functions of his storytelling may shift over the time it takes to tell the tale. Thus this analytic tool allows one to examine how children move back and forth across boundaries within the telling of a story.

INTERNAL AND EXTERNAL LANDSCAPES

One of the most powerful distinctions made through narrative is that of internal and external landscape, described best in the work of Jerome Bruner.[27] Every narrative paints two landscapes, one of action and one of consciousness. These two landscapes can inform one another, that is, overlap—or the author can stick pretty much to one of the landscapes. Contrast, for instance, James Joyce's *Ulysses* with Daniel Defoe's *Moll Flanders.*[28]

Young children tend to tell stories that describe the landscape of action, for example, "Once she came to my house and we hid some cookies. We played together. And then she went home." As they get older, children are more likely to talk about the landscape of consciousness, as in this piece of a narrative told by a ten-year-old boy about his friend: "Sometimes he'll feel sorry because he misses his grandfather. I think he was four when his grandfather passed away. He really liked him. He misses him."

But developmental differences along this dimension are not that simple, because in addition to a shift from internal to external landscape between the ages of four and ten, we also see a shift in the amount of flux within a story. From the time a child is about three until somewhere between the ages of eight and twelve (depending on cultural forces and the kind of schooling experience a child has), he is likely to play around with those two landscapes as he tells a story. Younger children slide back and forth between the two realms, finding out not only what is possible to convey in each landscape, but also how far they can go in manipulating the relationship between them. Older children stick more to one type or another, and to the extent that they are concerned with these forms, they do not visibly play with the possibilities while constructing narratives.

LIVED WORLD VERSUS IMAGINED WORLD

A second contrast children explore in their stories is the line between fact and fiction. We are used to this tension or contrast in the work of adult writers. Philip Roth is one shining example; note his coy novel *The Facts*, which is his way of toying with his readers who think they can figure out which parts of his novel are autobiographical and which are "pure fiction."[29] But the distinction is neither obvious nor static. Though research methods often push us toward creating straightforward dichotomies, fact and fiction are two ends of a continuum. Young children do not simply explore the line between fact and fiction. They also explore the dynamic boundary between everyday experience and fantasy.

Children often blend what has happened with what might have happened, or with what they are afraid or wish could happen. The two most obvious forms of this are when children tell an autobiographical story but insert fantasy and when they tell made-up stories and weave in actual things they have experienced. There are two kinds of experience they can draw on: direct experiences they have had, and experiences they have encountered through other narratives. In this way the narratives they construct give them a chance to integrate three different worlds of experience—the directly experienced, the heard about, and the imagined. Werner and other developmental psychologists have argued that early on, distinctions between domains of experience, real and imagined, aren't salient to children. But through narratives, children develop a sense of how and when boundaries between domains of thinking are operating.

We know that children borrow genres and styles from the stories they hear and read. But they also borrow experience, and often between the ages of four and ten their stories reflect their interest in exploring the relationships between their own experiences and the experiences of others. This lies at the core, after all, of the power of stories: the power to give us experiences beyond the immediate. It is an amplification of what Alexander Luria called the second world, the world afforded through symbols, particularly words.[30] When children borrow the experiences of others, it is one way that they share consciousness, which is a fundamental if not intrinsic aspect of what it is to be human.

In the following somewhat extended example, a child shifts back and forth between pure fantasy and information about another person's life (that of Jane Goodall), and information from his own direct experience. The story is recounted here in its entirety to give the reader a sense of what can be learned when children's stories are considered as processes that unfold in real time.

THE STORY OF JANE GOODALL

Long long ago, hundreds of scientists from all over the world were going to the jungle to study animals. But people kept on disappearing when they went to the jungle. Nobody knew why they were disappearing. Finally, the ruler of Zuubaarra told six very brave explorers to invent something to find out what the thing was that kept making people disappear. John, Jack, Bob, Bishop, Ariel and Matt were the scientists' names. For five years they built a machine. It flew above the jungle. It had a sensor that took pictures of any sights of life. Finally on April 23, they sent the machine on its mission. Eventually one whole year passed and the machine came back. They looked at all the pictures. All of them were of birds, tigers, and jaguars, except for one. It looked like a hairy human and it walked on two legs just like a human. So the six scientists decided to invent a trap and go to the jungle. It took them over one year to finish the trap. The scientists went to the jungle with the trap. Time passed, and eventually they made it to the jungle. The scientists waited in the jungle for the weird man-like animal to get trapped in the trap. The scientists waited all day and all night. In the morning when the scientists woke up the animal was trapped in the trap. The scientists were so amazed. At first they didn't know what to do. The scientists decided somehow they had to get the cage with the monkey in it into their boat. So all six of them grabbed onto the bars. They lifted and lifted and they got it up into the air and boom! They got it into the boat and luckily the boat didn't break. The six scientists jumped into the boat. The scientists started rowing the boat. After three hours they made it home. They pulled the cage out of the boat. The scientists dragged the cage into the lab. The scientists

> ran lots of tests. They put wires all over the thing. They ran a stress test. But after a couple of weeks something bad was happening to the scientists. They were throwing up and getting bad bloody noses, and much more. They decided to go to a doctor. It turned out they had gotten a disease from the jungle. They had to stay in the hospital. They never lived to find out what the thing was. 50 years passed. Things changed. But there was one lady who remembered those six scientists as heroes. Her name was Jane Goodall, and she wanted to go to the jungle and find out what those things were. She thought about if she should go or not. And there were reasons she shouldn't and there were reasons she should. But after all it wouldn't be too bad, so she decided to go. She packed up her bag with food and drinks and medicine. She rented a canoe and went to the jungle. She was exploring the jungle and going to all different places. Finally she got to this little cave-ish like thing that was made out of sticks and leaves. She went inside the cave. There were those things that nobody knew what they were. At first she was a little scared by them. Then the things jumped on her and they started petting her and hugging her. She noticed they weren't scary. So she started going farther into the cave. In the back of the cave there were all these old people that were trapped in there as slaves. She got the people up and helped them out of the cave. The monkeys started following her but then when she went out of the cave they stopped. She helped the people go back through the jungle. They got in her boat and they went home. She let the people out. She decided that she wanted to keep on going back to the jungle. She studied the things and decided that they weren't anything like humans except for their intellect. She named the things Chimpanzees. And that's the story of Jane Goodall.

In this story the author explicitly combines some factual material (Jane Goodall) with a completely imagined scenario about explorers in a jungle. But several other kinds of genres and texts are borrowed and integrated into the story. This author had heard a sibling reading the novel *Congo* out loud, and clearly took some strands regarding a dangerous hidden colony of apes, as well as the idea of a disease (probably the Ebola virus, which had interested this child greatly) carried back from the jungle. He may also have borrowed some of the plot of *Curious George* when describing the monkeys being carried in a cage with sticks and rowed in a boat.

INVENTED VERSUS BORROWED FORMS

Children often move back and forth within one story between a kind of free-form exploration of language and language play, and the use of forms he or she has heard in other people's stories (written and spoken). In the following example, a six-year-old boy wrote a story over a period of several days, in school. Details of how he came to write the story help the researcher understand what the form and content of the story itself can tell us about narratives. The little boy who wrote the story had a favorite book during the year called *The Paper Dragon,* which is about a Chinese artist who fights a dragon.[31] He had been reading the book one to four times a week over a period of several months. The book had a powerful influence on the story he created.

> *THE DRAGON PEOPLE*
> A long time ago there lived a young painter. His favorite thing to do was painting dragons. He was the best painter in the village. It seemed to the other people in the village that he painted all day. His favorite thing to paint were dragons. But one day a little boy came up to him and said "Will you paint a portrait of me?" "Sure" the painter said.
>
> So the painter started painting the little boy. Then the little boy heard his mother calling him for dinner.
>
> Since the boy was gone the painter started turning the boy's painting into a dragon. Suddenly the painting started moving. Then the dragon stepped out of the painting and started walking. More and more creatures stepped out of his paintings. Then the little boy came running back. The minute the boy saw the creatures he turned into

one of the creatures. The painter ran home. Finally he got home. He gasped and told his parents the story of his paintings.

Then his mom said "There is a legend that sounds like your story. A long time ago there was a young painter. He painted a half-boy, half-dragon that came to life. He tried everything to make him disappear. Finally he gave them love and they disappeared. The only way to make the creatures come back is to paint the same picture.

After listening to his mother's story, the painter ran back to his hill where he was painting. Before he knew it, sure enough, there were the creatures. So the painter tried to be nice to the creatures but he did not make them disappear. The reason he couldn't make the creatures disappear was because the creatures were not from the boy's picture but from the old legend. He had made them reappear through his painting.

It seemed to the painter that there were more creatures than the boy creature. Finally the painter ran home.

He screamed "MOM, DAD, WHERE ARE YOU?" There was no answer. So he went to his neighbors. He looked around. His neighbors weren't there either. Before he knew it he had gone to every house in the village. No one was in their house.

He went back to his hill. It seemed like there were more creatures than there were before. Then he saw one with hair just like his mom. He thought and thought. If there was a creature that looked like his mother and she wasn't home that could mean only one thing. She had turned into one of the creatures. And so had everyone else in the village.

He took the painting of the boy out of his pocket. He started writing a poem called *Dragons Play and Dance and Have Fun.* He went home. He got a rope out of his father's chest. He ran back to his hill. He tied the rope to the poem. He threw the poem over to where the creatures were. One of the creatures looked at the poem. Then some more and more came to look at the poem. Finally all the creatures came and read the poem.

The poem:
Play and dance,
Have fun and love,
Clouds drift by,
And birds fly.

The creatures started turning back into humans because the creatures remembered that they were loved before.

Then the painter and his mom and the boy and everybody else went back to the village.

The end.

One remarkable feature of this story is that it reveals so clearly the way in which young storytellers explore the very idea of genres and text in their stories. This story is about a painter who represents reality visually. It also contains a legend, an autobiographical account of what had happened (when the painter told his parents the story of his paintings), and a poem. In other words, it not only borrows from another text; it also uses the narrative form to explore kinds of text and the boundaries between texts. *The Dragon People* deals quite explicitly with the boundary between representations and the things represented when it explores the idea that a picture can come to life, and that a remembered story might affect current reality.

The story is long and complex. Though there is a clear plight, which is resolved, there are several twists and turns to the story, and some of them are confusing. On one level of analysis, the story simply reflects an incomplete command over the formal aspects of a narrative. It illustrates the ways in which six-year-olds do not yet adhere to a linear form for their stories. But on another level, it shows the purpose that storytelling has for this six-year-old. For instance, in the story the painter suddenly runs home to his mother and father, which seems unusual for an adult, and one cannot help but wonder if the author has mixed up the characters of the boy and the painter—in a sense, become lost in his own text. While this possible mistake leads to confusion for the reader, it also shows that storytelling is still, for this child, a dynamic form of play. What he is imagining and feeling as he tells the story is more salient to him than his ongoing sense of what his audience is hearing or understanding. The line between story as finished text and story as creative process is movable at best for young authors. Importantly, then, while some aspects of stories like this suggest immature command over narrative form—incomprehensible jumps in time, location, perspective, or character; ellipses; or abrupt changes in plot—these same features reflect what the story is doing for the child at that time. The story as text reveals certain aspects of the child's narrative ability, whereas the story as process shows what narrative "problems" the child is exploring, and how he makes sense of a range of influences on his inner life.

OPAQUE AND TRANSPARENT LANGUAGE

Much of the time that children are telling stories, particularly autobiographical stories, they use language transparently. That is, the language is not interesting or important in and of itself, but is a vehicle for communicating about events. But there are moments within a story where children will sometimes begin using language more opaquely. The language itself becomes part of what is important, meaningful, or pleasurable about the story. Consider the opening lines of the following story told by a five-year-old to her younger cousin. What begins as a fairly traditional story ("Once a long long time"), shifts by the second sentence. Something about the phrase or sound of teensy weensy grabs the narrator's attention. The sounds of the words suddenly become as salient as the story she is creating.

> Once a long long time, there was a teensy weensy girl. And she had a teensy weensy baby mousy. They lived in the woods, in a teensy teensy teensy housey.

As I have shown elsewhere, children between the ages of four and nine are often quite sensitive to the language used in the stories they hear. When they hear works by authors such as T. S. Eliot, William Faulkner, and Emily Dickinson, the work they create within the next twenty-four hours often contains language and style borrowed from those authors. Alyssa McCabe has shown that children who are exposed to a range of genres and techniques from other cultures use a wider range of storytelling language in their own stories.[32] But even without such influences, children commonly begin telling a story to narrate their play, or accompany a drawing, or recount an experience, but midway through the story, their interest shifts from plot to language. Take the following story, for example, told by a three-year-old to her mother: "The guys who went up the steep nicken and then he fell down and hurt his nicken on the schnocks of the nicks."

In examples such as this, the child may find ways to continue the plot while exploring language itself—by using alliteration, rhyming, repetition, changes in rhythm, and punning, to name just a few techniques. They may also drop the plot and get lost in language play, sometimes never returning to finish the story. How they balance opaque and transparent uses of language may depend on the storytelling situation as much as on the individual child or her stage of development.

SELF VERSUS OTHER

Finally, there is the dimension of self versus other. In the following story, dictated by a four-year-old boy, the storyteller seems to vacillate between putting his friend at the center of the narrative and putting himself in this important role.

> Carter plays with me, and he talks with me. And he plays with me at home. And he plays . . . Carter, well, plays sandbox with me . . . and he said, "You can come to my party and whack my piñata." And he goes whacking hard. But yesterday there was a piñata and I whacked it hard and all the candies came out. Yesterday was Carter's birthday

and I saw a sack of piñata and I whacked it. We had the birthday party at school.

One of the most powerful capabilities that narratives give us is the chance to think from someone else's perspective (whether we are creating or hearing a narrative). The ability to tell stories about other people, and eventually to tell stories from the perspective of other people, is a vital path to imagining the consciousness of others. The narratives of very young storytellers rarely include the perspective of others. During the first ten years of life this ability emerges, though researchers don't yet know why some people become good at it and others do not. It is apparent, however, that in the early years children experiment with the relationship of self and other—and stories give them a perfect medium for shifting back and forth as they try out perspective.

It should be apparent by now that most stories written or told by young children feature bits and pieces of each of these themes, even if only one at a time is dominant. In each example it would have been tempting to demonstrate the ways in which the other dimensions were also at work. To get the full picture of the mind behind the story, we need to track shifts along all five dimensions as a story unfolds, and to see how the changes in each relate to changes in the others.

My students and I have been coding children's stories, utterance by utterance, and giving each utterance a value of 1, 2, or 3. The three numbers represent values on an ordinal scale, and measure increasing levels of intensity on each of these dimensions. For instance, a child might include an utterance that was clearly transparent, clearly opaque (metaphor, pun, alliteration), or something in-between. Similarly, a child might describe an event that was obviously autobiographical, quite fantastical, or plausible fiction. While other researchers may come up with a different scale, or may disagree on the specific values we assigned to certain parts of a story, our initial goal was simply to see if one could chart a range of dynamics at work within a story. Examined together, such dynamics might give a visual image of the complexity, change, and mental activity that occurs with storytelling.

Looking at stories this way enables us to find out which dimensions are salient at given points of development, under various storytelling conditions, or for a particular child. It allows us to look for patterns and general principles that reveal how children think, but it retains the lively nature of storytelling. Research using this approach will show us whether the amount of oscillation within a story—that is, of switching back and forth between modes and interests—changes as a function of development. Perhaps there is more oscillation on all five dimensions in the stories and play narratives of four-year-old children than in those of seven-year-olds. But it would be equally interesting to find that the sources of oscillation change with development. Perhaps younger children explore the boundaries between fact and fiction and older children more frequently use stories to explore the boundaries between forms of storytelling.

This approach has implications beyond storytelling. It may shed light on the more general question of how children's spheres of experience change with development. A wide range of research on topics such as conceptual development, early language acquisition, emotional development, and interpersonal relationships suggests that over time children draw firmer and firmer boundaries between types of experience. For instance, between the ages of two and five children make increasingly clear, stable distinctions between language and its referents, self and other, fact and fiction, inanimate and animate objects, play and work, and scientific and magical explanations. The oscillations apparent in the stories and play of young children reflect their curiosity about spheres of experience, and the boundaries that define them. Perhaps these explorations decrease as the spheres that shape and define their experiences become more differentiated, and the boundaries between those spheres become firmer—and possibly because of that, less interesting to children.

While two- to five-year-old children use story and play to express highly personal and idiosyncratic interpretations of the world, by the time children are six or seven they delineate and interpret their daily experiences in accordance with their culture. That is, their interpretations of what is work, what is play, what is an acceptable explanation for events, and so on, are increasingly likely to match those of others around them. By the time most children are six or so, not only are the boundaries between spheres firmer and more stable, but the spheres themselves are also more embedded in social conventions.

As children leave early childhood, they become more self-conscious, attuned to the needs and expectations of others, and oriented toward shared rule systems. During this same period, magical thinking both decreases and becomes less explicit.[33] The frequency and pervasiveness of play decreases as well, and the rules that govern play become increasingly stable and conventional. In other words, checkers and baseball tend to replace pretend play.[34] Storytelling becomes more strictly a means of self-presentation and communication, and less a form of play and improvisation. Shifts between spheres of experience become more subtle, controlled, and private. Looking at the stories and play older children do engage in, it is clear that the kind of dynamic flux characteristic of young children wanes with development.

One can see in young children's play, and then in their stories, that the very way they approach everyday life differs fundamentally from most adults. It is not simply that the kinds of rules children apply to experience, or their level of logic and abstract thinking, are different from the rules that govern adult experience: children have a different way of psychologically carving up the world. It is said that Jorge Luis Borges used to carefully stand all his books on their spines at night, so the words wouldn't fall out while he slept. This suggests that what is true for a few adults is probably characteristic of most children—the boundaries that separate kinds of experience are flexible and permeable. Many seemingly prosaic experiences of everyday life invite active, lively construal.

To learn more about how such abilities function in a fluctuating, imaginative, playful, and emotional child, we need better tools for looking at children in action, in real settings. Though play, narrative, and the orientations that accompany such activities have been central to my own interests, narratives are not the only way to learn about how children construct meanings and experience their world. Figuring out how to study children is as pressing a question today as it was when Piaget first began to devise his methods.

4 Toward a More Complete Understanding of Children

While researchers have done a superb job of pinpointing specific skills and measuring the effect of certain experiences on later development, they have been less successful, or interested, in grasping the experiences of early childhood. Some of this has to do with a tension in the field regarding the nature of psychological research. Should research only concern itself with isolating causes and effects? Can research be rigorous and trustworthy when it ventures to interpret observational data, or to take a person's accounts of their own experience seriously? The tension gets played out on two levels: what should be studied, and how should it be studied?

Many argue that you can only study behaviors; for example, you can't know what a child imagines about her mother, but you can see what she does when the mother leaves the room. In recent years, however, there has been increasing interest in children's representations of experience—their pictures, stories, and dramatizations. This interest is based on the realization that such representations are clues to the child's mental life, and provide the child with a powerful set of guides for how to behave in the world. Thus, researchers have expanded their notions of what should be studied to include children's art, stories, and play.

Meanwhile, there has been a corresponding shift in how to do developmental research. Some have argued that the usual experimental approaches do not capture all that is of interest when investigating children's development. Isolating variables and describing general clusters of behaviors leave too much out of the picture.

Some, like me, would argue that we need both experimental methods that isolate variables, and more naturalistic methods that identify the more multilayered, emergent characteristics of young children in real-world settings.

Phenomena don't stand still, and neither do children. Because we can, to some extent, see children thinking, feeling, and behaving in real time and space, the flow of their mental activity offers clues about what is really going on inside their minds. In arguing that experiments and quantitative methods fall short when it comes to understanding individual psychology, and change over time, the cultural psychologist Michael Cole quotes novelist Walker Percy: "There is a secret about the scientific method which every scientist knows and takes as a matter of course, but which the layman does not know . . . The secret is this: Science cannot utter a single word about the individual molecule, thing, or creature in so far as it is an individual but only in so far as it is like other individuals." Cole comments, "Applied to psychology, the discipline which studies individual behavior and consciousness, this limitation of the scientific method is particularly disheartening."[1] I would add to Cole's commentary that when it comes to understanding the young child, whose consciousness holds clues to our adult consciousness and yet seems to be so qualitatively distinct from it, this problem is ever more pressing.

One solution to the shortcoming that Cole and Percy identify is to enrich our scientific methods. When it comes to trying to understand children's minds, we have to get at least a little closer to understanding their experience. In order to do this, two things are required: much closer descriptions of what they do and how they do it in real life, and better attempts to characterize their thoughts, feelings, and ways of construing their world. In other words, we need more detailed accounts of children engaged in everyday activities. Those accounts need to include the social and physical context of their behavior. Moreover, two kinds of accounts are called for—conventional descriptions very much like ethnographies and naturalistic records of behavior, as well as attempts to find out what the child thinks and feels. In order to construct such characterizations, we need to pay a great deal of attention to individual experience. It is only by getting some more specific information on children in all their complexity, and using this to begin to construct an understanding of their experience, that we will have a fuller picture of their mental lives. In the end, even the other goals, such as determining outcomes, will only be accurate if they rest on richer, more precise descriptions.

The living, breathing child encountering the world is often different than the one captured in the isolated situations and moments constructed in experiments. For the past seventy years or so, research has identified children's thoughts and actions from the outside looking in. The observer records what the child does and says, and tries as hard as possible to keep distance between him- or herself and the subject. I call this the third-person approach. Take for example, the following description from a current study of young children's ability to discriminate and compare sizes of things. The researchers were interested in finding out whether children under the age of four could tell when one dowel was larger or smaller than one they had seen earlier. I quote here from one small section of the article: "Each infant was tested in a single session lasting approximately 10 minutes. A parent held the infant on his or her lap, 2 feet from the opening of the stage in a small booth. During the procedure, the parent wore a blindfold and was asked to avoid interaction with the infant. (Then the children were taken through three phases of the test: familiarization, habituation, and the test itself.) Looking times were recorded on a computer by an observer who watched the infant's looking behavior on a monitor behind the stage during the experiment."[2] The study, well designed and carefully carried out, yielded valuable information about the limitations of the infant's ability to discriminate between different sizes, and shows that even though they know more than we used to think they knew, they don't think as adults do. But some of the very characteristics that make this study seem strong from one perspective limit its value from another perspective. The experimenters asked parents to wear blindfolds so that any claims about the infant's ability to judge the size of the dowels was based as purely as possible on the infant's individual skill, rather than some influence of the parent. The blindfold made the assessment of the infant more pure. As a wealth of research has shown, however, infant's abilities emerge in an "impure" context. Parents do cue their children, and children learn from such cueing. Similarly, it is rare in everyday life for a child to be exposed to an experience for an isolated ten minutes. Development takes place over time. So two of the features of this study that seem to strengthen it in conventional social scientific terms weaken it in terms of its relation to the way such cognitive abilities emerge in real life. But along with these methodological features the study exemplifies a pervasive theme of contemporary research: an underlying preoccupation with competence as the key measure of what children are like.

Take, for example, the following sentence that introduces a piece of excellent research in a current journal: "Recent years have witnessed a growing body of evidence supporting the impressive competencies of young children in reasoning about the mind and mental states."[3] Our focus on competencies has yielded valuable and usable knowledge about what young children can do, how much they can learn, and how we might best facilitate such learning. It has dramatically altered our view of young children, giving us a much more impressive estimation of their skills and abilities, particularly their sense-making skills. We have learned that although children may not always be able to explain their knowledge the way that we can, their knowledge may nonetheless be organized, generative, and complex. Children seem able to think and solve problems in ways we never would have expected even ten years ago. But the focus on skills has nourished a preoccupation with outcomes.

A common emphasis of recent research, and public interest in childhood, has been questions of cause and effect. For instance, one central topic of burning interest to researchers, parents, and policy makers concerns the relative influence of genetics, parental input, and peers in shaping a child's prospects. That is, what are the predominant forces that determine who is smart and who is not, who will be well socialized and who will be a criminal?[4] The researchers who investigate these questions approach the topic from different perspectives: measurement, cognition, clinical psychology, genetics, and social psychology. In his recent book *The Myth of the First Three Years,* John T. Bruer argues against the popular notion that a child's outcome is set within the first three years of life. He shows how little we still know about neurological development in infancy and childhood, and at the same time, how much we know about the powerful influences of later experience, not only on behavior but also on the structure of the brain itself.[5]

Another issue of great concern to researchers and educators is educational methods and their success. What methods ensure that all children will learn to read? How many students can one teacher teach in a classroom if all children are to end the year with certain skills or knowledge?

Both these controversies involve describing the child's behavior from the outside, and ascertaining exactly what we can do to influence a good outcome in as many children as possible. But there are some important drawbacks to this impressive and huge body of diverse research. One limitation is the assumption that the human organism is predictable enough to control (if we use technique X when children are three, then they will all be able to do Y when they are eight). Because children are by definition in transition, they are much more unpredictable and their interactions too complex to control in the way some research would lead you to expect. Hence large-scale studies that attempt to identify such cause and effect have tended to hedge their bets by taking too many sides. The most striking example of this is the research on the effects of day care on young children. Every time a study seems to have found the one clear way in which a certain kind of care in infancy or toddlerhood leads to a specific outcome in preschool or school-age children, it turns out that individual differences account for as much variation as the central variable.[6] It seems unlikely that we will come up with models of education or child rearing that could ensure that all children will have certain attributes, or lack certain undesirable qualities. In addition, this direction has led us increasingly away from thinking about how the world looks and feels from the child's perspective.

The third-person approach, moreover, has still not answered our most fundamental questions about children's mental development. Recently one hundred developmental psychologists from all over the world gathered in a meeting room to debate various interpretations of a section from one of Piaget's best-known and richest books, *Play, Dreams, and Imitation in Childhood.*[7] In the middle of a fairly technical and somewhat obscure debate regarding the nature of an infant's ability to symbolize, one of the researchers, John Flavell, said, "I still would like to know whether, when the mother leaves the room, a nine-months-old baby has an image of his mother in his head. I would like to know what the baby's mental life is like."[8] This statement is startling in its simplicity. Flavell's comment cuts right to the core of the matter and suggests that we have yet to fully answer our most basic questions about development. But to address this question we may need to try to decipher the world from the child's perspective. In other words, developmental psychologists and educators need periodically to take a first-person approach to understanding young children.

Recently a young colleague was talking with me about research on the development of the self. I mentioned some of the more inchoate feelings and strivings that William James identified in his classic work on the topic, over a hundred years ago.[9] I suggested to my colleague that these strivings and inner musings needed to be more fully understood, but that in order to understand them, one would have to capture them as they unfold in everyday interactions. My colleague replied, "If I can't bottle it and bring it into the lab, I'm not interested in it." I believe that his view has become predominant among research psychologists, and that if we all adopt it we will eventually be studying things that have nothing to do with psychology. In the middle of his career in research, the highly regarded experimental psychologist Sigmund Koch had something of an epiphany that changed the direction of his work. He argued that psychology had become too rigid in its methodologies and in so doing excluded the very phenomena of most interest. He termed his colleagues' preoccupation with certain research approaches "methodological fetishism," and urged the field to be more open and creative in its methods of inquiry. In particular, he suggested that researchers employ "indigenous methodologies"—that is, whatever methods most closely capture and reflect a given kind of phenomena.[10]

What Heinz Werner argued all those years ago is still true, and still underappreciated in the world of developmental research: to understand the child's mind, one must contend with the child in a world of everyday real-life objects, events, and people.[11] Doing so in part involves thinking about children's everyday lives—the rhythms, idiosyncrasies, and textures of their actual experience. Researchers have, for a long time, tried to document the conditions of children's lives, and understand development within such an ecological framework (sometimes this framework is even referred to as the "ecology of childhood").[12] But the suggestion here goes beyond a need to document differences in culture, economies, and cohort.

THE VALUE OF DESCRIPTION

The first step is a deceptively simple one. We need more close descriptions of children in their everyday lives. Meticulous observation and description as a respected method has all but died in developmental psychology. The last big studies that involved careful descriptions of children over time were recounted in Roger Brown's *A First Language* in 1973, and Uri Bronfenbrenner's *Two Worlds of Childhood* in 1970. Roger Brown tracked three children in Cambridge, Massachusetts, as they learned to talk, and though his account contained little biographical information about his three young subjects, his record did show their first attempts at language in very full detail.[13]

Uri Bronfenbrenner described children in the Soviet Union and the United States in order to show that a child's development could not be understood apart from his or her culture.[14] Though the two works had very different scientific foci, and stemmed from disparate theoretical frameworks, they shared an emphasis on descriptions of children in their real-life situations. Over the years, now and then a book or study will appear that centers on careful descriptions of children in their natural settings. Peggy Miller and Wendy Haight, for instance, wrote a book on children's play that offered detailed descriptions of children playing at home with their mothers.[15] Similarly, Marilyn Shatz undertook an analysis of her grandchild's play over time.[16] Judy Dunn's research, too, focuses on children's play and interactions in natural settings, and identifies how children use their everyday interactions to build skills and knowledge.[17] But studies such as these are few and far between, and rarely presented in the journals that provide most researchers with their frame of reference. These methods need to be used again and again, for all kinds of topics within developmental psychology.

At least two kinds of descriptive data would contribute invaluably to our understanding of child development. First, we need more descriptions of more children in a wider range of settings. To take one small example: Researchers have recently found that children are more able than we previously thought to solve certain kinds of logical problems, such as syllogisms. It seems that when children are invited to think syllogistically in an imaginary framework, they do much better. Cassandra Richards and Jennifer Sanderson presented two-year-old children with the following propositions and question: All fish live in trees. Tot is a fish. Does tot live in a tree? Research in the past has found that toddlers are likely to answer such syllogistic questions not in terms of the logical relations of the propositions, but in terms of what they know: fish don't live in trees. When Richards and Sanderson told their young subjects to imagine a special faraway planet where fish live in trees, however, two-year-olds could solve the syllogisms.[18] Research such as this suggests, rather strongly, that a child's framework for interpreting an activity is important. But to be as informative as possible, such results need to be understood in a larger picture—when do children encounter logical problems in everyday life? How likely are they to adopt an imaginary orientation? What other internal and external forces shape their response to a given situation? This expanded view might enable us to know not only what children can do under highly constrained crafted situations, but also what they will do in the range of situations they usually encounter. We need richer canvasses within which to place our more focused, fine-grained results. In particular, we should record children with video cameras in everyday settings, fit them with unobtrusive audio recording devices, and include data collected through old-fashioned observation and field notes.

But a second kind of description is needed as well. Ethnographies of childhood provide us with a broad canvas for understanding specific processes. But psychologists often assume that they can then go right from the ethnography to the experiment, or conversely that they can simply draw on ethnographies to help shade or fill in the results of their experiments. We also need close descriptions of children as they engage in various tasks—moment-by-moment records of a child's words, facial expressions, and gestures such as those relied on by Piaget and Vygotsky.[19] In fact, today a number of studies are being conducted that record children over time. This approach is called microgenetic because the researchers attempt to identify change as it happens (how a child's thinking is affected by trying a task several times, for instance). Microgenetic studies specify the psychological steps that children take in solving a problem, or infer changes in thinking from one attempt at a task to another. Implicit in such work is the understanding that children's thinking unfolds in real time and that their actions and words offer a window onto their thoughts. Take, for example, Dan Stern's close analysis of mothers and infants playing. The concept of attunement and parent-child mismatch that resulted from that work has had a huge influence on our understanding of early mother-child interaction. Those data depended on watching mothers and babies over time. The advent of video data, and the technology to analyze small segments of behavior, have made this kind of close observation an even more powerful method of research.[20]

But it is not enough to simply chart the myriad schedules, life events, and behaviors in real settings and in real time. We also need a better understanding of how children think and feel within these settings. Part of what we need is to pay more serious and more discerning attention to what children tell us about their experience of everyday life. The luminary educator Deborah Meier, in her book *In Schools We Trust,* explains what keeps her so interested in schools and teaching: "I'm still as fascinated as I was the day I began teaching in Beulah Shoesmith School on Chicago's South Side by the details of how each and every child learns to put together the meaning of his or her own world."[21] What makes this statement striking is that it is the exception, not the rule, for a teacher to put this task, this question, at the forefront of her teaching. In her book *Tell Me More,* Eleanor Duckworth describes the ways in which teachers can guide their own practices by finding out what a given learner is experiencing.[22] Though framed as advice to teachers, her approach reminds us that paying attention to what a child is experiencing is a valuable source of information. Not coincidentally, Duckworth, a professor of education at Harvard, worked as Piaget's translator for many years, and has written extensively on the implications of Piaget's theory for teaching. What educators such as Meier and Duckworth propose for teachers is good advice for psychological researchers as well. They are urging us to focus on how a given child, age level, or group of children put together the meaning of their worlds. One way to achieve such understanding is for psychologists and teachers to collaborate more.

Another valuable source of such information comes from children themselves, when they tell us about their experiences. As I mentioned in Chapter 3, Robert Emde and his colleagues have developed a specific research tool, the MacArthur Story Stem, for eliciting stories from children that express their feelings about various life events.[23] This is one example of how we might take what children say about their lives more seriously.

LISTENING TO CHILDREN

Children don't begin life talking, but by the time they are three years old, words, sentences, monologues, and dialogues are an essential part of their everyday experience. Language becomes central to what it means to be human. Charles Darwin, who kept a diary of his own child, was one of the first scientists to characterize the baby as a biological creature, defined by her appetites, reflexes, and physical characteristics.[24] In support of this biological view, most research has shown that certain abilities and activities—such as walking, talking, planning, problem solving, and some form of reciprocity in relationships—develop to some degree almost no matter what happens to a child (barring extreme cases of neglect and abuse). Of these, perhaps the most dramatic and transformative is the use of language.

What catapults the human being from a basically biological state into the world of thinking, feeling interactions that seem to define us as a species? Many would now argue that it is our symbolic capacity, most specifically our ability to use language, that lifts us out of a biological state and into the world of culture. Whereas the baby's mental development is tied to immediate forces (her own appetites, actions, and responses, and proximal features of the environment), the three-year-old child energetically brings her symbolic processes to bear on everything she encounters in herself and in the world around her. Several important books in recent years have explored this phenomenon in far greater depth than I will (*Origins of the Modern Mind* and *The Cultural Origins of Human Cognition* to name two new ones, and of course Lev Vygotsky's classic *Thought and Language*).[25] My point here is not to trace the development of language, but instead to make a case for how central language is in providing a bridge from infancy to childhood. Once acquired, language begins to shape development, as well as mold the child's inner experience. Language does something else as well: it provides us with an invaluable window into children's inner lives.

Contrast, for instance, a toddler room at a day care center with a preschool room at the same center. I watch two little boys, about twenty-two months old, riding. The first one, Chris, wanders over and gets on a little plastic motorcycle-type vehicle, and begins riding it around. The pretend-play aspect of his activity is fleeting, often completely overshadowed by the motoric activities—using his feet to push along his motorcycle. He makes a low buzzing noise, probably of the motorcycle's engine. But his sounds are unelaborated, and again, seem as if they are there for the way they feel rather than the way they embellish or add to a scenario or pretense. The other little boy, Matthew, notices what Chris is doing, gets up from his chair at the clay table with great purpose, and walks over to get on the other little plastic motorcycle vehicle. He begins pushing his motorcycle around, following Chris. They buzz around the room for quite a time, making an imaginary route. There is little conversation, or development of the pretense. Instead the energy seems fully placed on the riding itself. At some point the first little boy stops, the second little boy runs into him, and the two vehicles fall over, one child toppling onto the other. This part of the episode happens silently and sluggishly. The little boys fall on top of one another with almost no expression on their faces, and it takes them almost sixty seconds to disentangle and each get back up on their bikes, which they only manage successfully when an adult comes over and hauls one off of the other one. It's an often silent and blurry time of life, when one activity blends into another, when the body often dominates or stands in for the mind. Watching these children, and comparing them to their three- and four-year-old counterparts in the room down the hall, one is struck by the tremendous differences in the way they play. And if one had to name a single characteristic on which they differ most, or most importantly, it would be language.

Day care professionals can regularly be heard admonishing

young children to "use their words." A little boy knocks another child over in his effort to get hold of the doll that he wants. The fallen child begins to sob, and the teacher says, "Okay, Milo, use your words. Tell Alexis you didn't like being knocked down." Here what the teacher means is replace action with words, and she means these words to be used between children to negotiate conflict—say your feelings and then you won't need to hit or grab. But that is only one way a toddler begins to use his words. More importantly, and dramatically, he begins to use his words to create a second, symbolic level of experience. This level allows him to plan, to imagine, to develop thoughts and scenarios, to communicate more than needs, and to transform both himself and his world.

Margaret Donaldson has argued that planning is what makes us distinct from other primates. Certainly planning is a symbolic, not to mention linguistic, activity. The idea that language is central to higher-order thinking has pervaded contemporary work on cognitive development.[26] Several different models have focused on the idea that in one way or another the child's increasing ability to function symbolically is key to his increasing intellectual power. For instance, the developmental psychologists John Flavell and Ann Brown introduced the idea that it is thinking about thinking that distinguishes older children from younger children.[27] This too, like planning, is at heart a linguistic activity. But language affords children other, less rational processes that are equally essential to the way they experience themselves and the world around them. Language exponentially expands and complicates the child's experience of herself and the world by giving her a range of ways to structure and reflect on her realities. Thus language affords us an essential window onto their inner worlds.

Sometimes children put their experiences into words that are so vivid that one cannot ignore the distinctiveness of their view nor the potency of life experience on a particular child's thinking and development. The following is a portion of something a nine-year-old boy wrote as his brother lay dying of cancer.

Based on a true story by C. M.

Chapter one: What would you do
My brother is dieing. Nothing could help him. Not plasma, not any kind of medicen. It is hopeless. What would you do if this happened to you. It may be hard. It may be touch, but be happy it isn't you. If our brother dies, be happy. It is better for him to die, then he won't be sufering.

Chapter 2: its ok
Its ok for you to cry. It won't make you look bad, it won't make you look stupid. Its better to let it out than hold it in. Nothing is wrong with crying. Its ok to show your sadness. Just don't show it to much. Just remember the good times. My brother was funny, so I remember the times he made me laugh. He was nice so I remember the times he did stuff for me and when he bought me presents.

Chapter 3: The pain for the child
If your child is dieing he may be in a lot of pain. But the suffring for a child with his brother is also painfull. Take it from me. I'm only 9 and I'll be 10 in May. My brother just might make it to see me 10. It is very painful for me. But god keeps on pulling off miracles. He almost died one day after school, but god puld off another one of his great miracles.

Luckily not all children go through events so dramatic or devastating. But that should not prevent us from realizing that all children do experience their world in vivid ways, and that they are often more capable of telling us about that experience than we give them credit for.

There are three ways to listen carefully to what children say. The first is simply to record what they say as they engage in various activities, the second is to record the language they use with one another, and the third is to ask questions and engage in open-ended conversations with them.

Often, as Vygotsky first demonstrated, children narrate their own activity. Vygotsky in fact claimed that they used language to guide action.[28] To the extent that this is true, listening to what they say as they solve tasks, play, and go about daily life is one way to find out how and what they are doing, as well as what they are feeling.

Recording the language that children use with one another can be difficult because it involves recording children so unobtrusively that they actually will go about their lives while being recorded. An excellent example of this is Gordon Wells's work in Bristol, England, in which he fitted each child with a small vest containing a microphone attached to a tape recorder so that he could record their everyday interactions with family members. It is also possible to set up recording devices in the corner of a day care center or nursery school.[29] This simple approach is not used often enough, even though sometimes what a child says to those around him offers valuable clues about not only what he is feeling or thinking, but also how his feelings and thinking shape one another.

In one example, recorded at the toddler room in a rural day care center, a toddler has just watched a little girl vomit all over the day care center floor. The little girl has been stripped down to her pink socks, and is getting cleaned up in the bathroom area. Another teacher is disinfecting the small plastic bike she was using when she threw up. The little boy, twenty-three months old, observes all this with solemn curiosity. After a little while he turns to the teacher and says, "My body feels better. My body does feel better. My body feels better. It feels better. My body DOES feel better." Finally the teacher looks up and replies, "That's good." Satisfied with her eventual acknowledgment, he returns to the sand table, where he had been playing with another child. What was going on inside his mind during this episode? One might guess that he was somehow linking what happened to the little girl to his own bodily state. He wanted to make it clear, to himself and his teacher, that he was okay—that he too hadn't gotten sick. He knew some comparison was in order (hence the "better" rather than "good," "healthy," or "well"). He needed verification that he had been heard, which is why he repeated it until the teacher responded. His strange litany of utterances doesn't fit into any of the theories of cognitive development that we currently work from in thinking about young children. Its tone and structure is urgent and insistent. Yet this urgency is what propels him into forging a powerful link between using words to mean and using them to do things (he describes how he feels, but he also makes himself feel better by announcing it to someone else). This kind of dynamic interaction between his impulses and his cognitive tools falls outside the realm of strictly rational views of early development, and can only be captured by seeing children in situations where their impulses and their cognitive tools collide.

The third approach, conversing with children, interestingly has its roots in Piaget's original method of inquiry but has received little serious attention in recent years. In his early experiments Piaget not only gave children tasks to solve (explaining, for instance, how a three-dimensional model of three mountains might look to a doll sitting on the other side of the model), but he also asked them to explain the answer they gave. He stressed the value of this kind of inquiry, and named it the "méthode clinique." The idea was to keep probing until you found out something about how the child viewed his own processes and/or the task, as well as his reasons for giving particular answers. As Piaget explained, "If we follow up each of the child's answers, and then, allowing him to take the lead, induce him to talk more and more freely, we shall gradually establish for every department of intelligence a method of clinical analysis analogous to that which has been adopted by psychiatrists as a means of diagnosis."[30] There are a handful of contemporary examples of this approach, described in Karen Bartsch and Henry Wellman's book *Children Talk about the Mind,* and Herbert Ginsburg's book *Entering the Child's Mind.*[31] Of course many contemporary psychologists ask children to explain why they have chosen a certain answer to a question, or solved a puzzle in a certain way. Asking children to explain their responses in experiments is a common practice and often requires the child to reflect on her own processes (the kind of metacognition I described in Chapter 2). But this is not the same as exploring the child's spontaneous interpretations of events, which reveal what she thinks about, and how. We need to revive this method.

TAKING PICTURES AND STORIES SERIOUSLY

In our culture at least, making pictures and telling stories are among children's favorite activities. Children are eager to draw and narrate, and their stories and pictures require a great deal of energy. These activities are not for the talented few, nor are children overly concerned with achievement as we think of it. Instead these seem to be intrinsically rewarding, meaningful ways for children to spend time. It is likely that this is because early in life drawing and storytelling are two primary means of thinking through experiences and communicating those experiences with others. Yet children's stories and art somehow have been sidelined as sources of insight into the child's thinking. In my own research, I have collected stories across a broad range of settings, including children's homes, schools, and playgrounds. In addition, I have interviewed children individually, seeking to elicit certain kinds of stories. For instance, in one recent study a student of mine, Alice Li, tape-recorded children between the ages of four and ten telling one another stories about friends while at school. The results were interesting because they gave us a picture of children spontaneously sharing certain kinds of information about one another in the form of stories. We followed up on this approach by taking children one at a time into a quiet room, getting into a conversation with them about their friendships and social lives, and finally asking them to tell us stories about one of those friends. These stories offered a great deal of information about the kinds of narratives young children construct, and what sources of information they use in constructing those narratives. For instance, younger children's stories were based almost entirely on shared experiences with friends, while ten-year-olds incorporated a fair amount of gossip and second-hand information. This suggested to us that over time children weave together different kinds of narrative material to reflect on their friends. In this case a more naturalistic, observational approach led to a more controlled study. The two sets of data were most interesting when considered together. These stories reveal an aspect of children's thoughts about one another that would be hard to access any other way.

I have also found, over the many years I have been collecting children's stories, that there are many kinds of stories (themes, forms, and processes) that are hard to capture in a lab. Motivation and context are so pivotal to what a child puts into a story, and to the storytelling itself, that one must be willing to take the inefficient approach of collecting them as they appear in a wide range of settings. I could not have collected the stories I have analyzed without the cooperation of many parents and teachers, nor could I have been attuned to this variety without having spent a great deal of time sitting in the corner of day care centers, playgrounds, nursery schools, and living rooms.

Whether the data are words, pictures, or a child's behavior, a key concern of this book has to do with how we take such evidence. In other words, what do a child's words, pictures, or behaviors tell us? These sorts of information can be used to draw certain conclusions about outcomes and abilities. But they can also tell us a great deal about the child's experience. The two goals are more connected than one might think: without thinking more carefully about the child's experience, the data on outcomes and abilities are not as useful as they might otherwise be. So the question becomes, how do we study children's experience?

CONSIDERING CHILDREN'S EXPERIENCE

Imagine a room with a wooden floor. In the middle of the room is a large pile of thick mud. Children, one at a time, are brought into the room and secretly taped. What does each child do? Are children of the same age more or less likely to do the same thing with the mud? Do boys behave one way, and girls another? As a researcher one has choices: Do I count the number of minutes it takes each child to start touching the mud? Do I decide ahead of time on three different levels of sophistication (swooshing your hands in the mud, building something with the mud, trying to figure out what the mud is made of), and code each child as being in one category or another? Another possibility is to describe step by step what each child does with the mud, and look for similar patterns among the children. Finally I might interpret each child's behavior in terms of what I think they are feeling. At the same time that I as the researcher have choices about how to make sense of such an experimental opportunity, the child who encounters the mud may have choices about what to do. One child may see the mud as in invitation to play. Another may see it as a challenge or test to be passed. Another child may look at it and fall into a daydream about past times at the beach. And finally there may be a child for whom the mud triggers a story, but without anyone else in the room to tell it to, she just sits there looking passive or disinterested.

My point is that all too often we forget that a basic question of developmental psychology is not what we can pull out of a child under certain conditions, but rather how different settings and situations elicit different kinds of responses from them. This question has to do with understanding how children approach a given setting (a place, an event, a conversation) and what aspects of that setting are salient to them. The seeds of such a focus are not new. The understanding that children's internal experience might be interesting dates back at least to the nineteenth century. In her historical account of nineteenth-century views of childhood, Carolyn Steedman argues that Goethe's character Mignon, from his book *Wilhelm Meister's Apprenticeship,* embodied the modern sense that children had what Steedman calls "interiority," or subjectivity.[32] Finding investigative methods to understand such interiority, and yet meet contemporary scientific standards, has proved somewhat elusive. But no matter how one might manage to suppress or ignore the child's subjectivity in the lab, it is hard to miss it in everyday life.

Once in a while a child does something that sharply reminds us that children's experience may be of a whole different order than ours, and that the child's day is filled with events that are not easily codified or captured by current models. A friend happened one day to walk by her three-year-old son's bedroom while he was playing inside. He was unaware of her, and was in the middle of enacting a scenario involving several characters planning a battle. There was a great deal of talk going on, with each character taking on a special voice and contributing to the plan. Suddenly the little boy looked up and saw his mother. Clearly taken aback that she had been watching, he said in a dignified, slightly put-out tone, "We want our privacy."

What do we make of this comment? From the outside looking in, one can describe the child's ability, at three, to plan an imaginary scenario. One might record his use of language and assess his vocabulary size, his grammatical complexity, and his ability to construct a narrative using several perspectives or characters. One might also speculate on his understanding of the boundary between real and not real, and look to see how his enactment of the characters reveals the distinctions he can make between his thoughts and the thoughts of others. But what does he feel and think as he plays? What does it mean to him to say to the adult, "We want our privacy"?

Now imagine a laboratory set up as a living room, containing comfortable furniture and some toys. A child has been brought in and asked to sit at a table containing some interesting objects. A friendly young woman sits across from him and begins to ask him some questions about which objects belong together and why. His answers and his actions with the objects may tell us a great deal about how he thinks about objects. He may touch them or even group them in terms of their color, or what they can do, or some other way in which they can be categorized. We might learn from this experiment what kind of a conceptual system the child uses at a certain age. We can also learn quite a bit about the kinds of mental strategies he uses. (If asked to remember objects from the table, will he say the names over and over again in his head? Will he group them into easily memorizable categories?) If asked to explain whether there are more cars or toys on the table, his answer will tell us something about how abstract his thinking is, and we might learn something about the kinds of rules he employs to solve problems. But what, we might ask, is he feeling and thinking in that moment, given that particular person and set of objects and questions? Why does he think he's in the room? How much is his mind on the task at hand? What actually excites or scares him about the situation?

Consider a slightly stranger and more jolting example. We probably all agree that when a four-month-old is confronted with a breast, he or she is likely to see it as an invitation to suck. The situation, as it were, elicits a pretty stable reaction across a broad range of four-month-olds—a reaction that can in fact tell us a lot about the inner life of the four-month-old. By contrast, confront a twenty-one-year-old adult with a breast and the range of reactions is bound to vary a lot. Some, perhaps many, will see it as a sexual opportunity (to act on or to fantasize about, but sexual nonetheless). Some may see it in other terms: a woman might compare it to her own breast, an artist might think of painting it, a doctor might think of the possible disease within it, and an author might be interested in remembering the situation to use in a later book. But what of the three- or four-year-old? The situation is not likely to elicit a purely sexual response in a preschooler, nor will it elicit the straightforward sucking response of a baby. It may elicit both kinds of responses, possibly in sequence, or even simultaneously. The ambiguity or multiplicity of the three-year-old's response tells us something about how he construes his encounters with everyday experiences—which we need to know more about. A good beginning question for any observation or study involving young children, then, is to ask what kinds of thoughts and impulses the situation might elicit in a given child (or age group). The answer to this question not only provides a backdrop for the interpretation of subsequent data, but also may provide clues about the complex and fluid quality of children's responses to a given experience.

In many of the examples I have presented so far, a striking feature is the way in which children shift their interpretation of a situation midstream, or reconstrue the same setting and objects in two different ways at two different times. This suggests that in order to get a real bead on children, we need to see them as moving among different kinds of thinking and activity. Recently I was sitting in a movie theater watching a documentary film about bird migration. A boy about four years old was sitting behind me on his mother's lap. Early on he was naming various birds and their behaviors. He was clearly a bright, articulate child who already knew a great deal about birds. He said, "That's a blue heron. Those two geese are fighting over a mate," and so on. At one point, a bird with a very long neck floated by on a lake, with his body completely submerged. Suddenly the boy called out in a somewhat anxious voice, "That bird's got no body!" His way of thinking had clearly slipped into a somewhat different realm, one of appearances and impossibilities, rather than the catalogue of information he had been previously drawing on. A little while later, the film showed a bird walking along in some very gooey mud. The little boy began to whisper "squish, squish, squish, squish." He was now narrating the film, focusing on sensations and the sound of words rather than the information being presented. One had to listen to this little boy for a full forty-five minutes to hear him move from one mode of response to another, and not one of those modes could accurately capture the child's mindset without the others. Recording his responses over time gave me a different view of his mind than I could have gotten in any given five-minute segment. But recording children over time will not in and of itself give us the full picture. The child researcher must also embrace rather than avoid the fact that each child's responses are determined by a range of factors, only some of which are easily visible to an observer.

Recently I watched a group of four- to six-year-olds in their school. They were seated on the floor in a circle, listening to their art teacher, who was sitting on a small chair at the head of the class. She was reminding them of the work they had begun in art class the week before—making small picture books about opposites. She then began to describe what they would do in today's art class. As she spoke, I watched the children's faces. One stared into space. Another carefully monitored the teacher's face. A third studied the face of the little girl sitting next to her. Suddenly one little boy enthusiastically threw his hand up in the air, eager to be called on. The teacher, delighted that someone had a question about her plans and the project she was introducing, called on him. "Yes, Ben. You have something to ask." He nodded energetically. "Can I go to the bathroom right now?" What was in his head had little to do with what was going on around him. Yet his thoughts, or in this case, sensations, had a dramatic influence on what he could do in the circle time, and what he might or might not internalize of the activities going on around him. The meaning of the event was quite different for him than for the other children and certainly far removed from the adult's construction of the activity. What was in Ben's mind had a great deal to do with the constraints of context. Naturally the teacher, who was in control, and therefore constraining the context, was not thinking about the concerns preoccupying Ben. The assumption that if the teacher is talking everyone is or should be "on the same page" may be a faulty one. The challenge for the researcher is to understand that what is on the child's mind may not neatly match what the context would suggest. Though the situation is not altogether different for adults (an adult could easily be thinking about having to use the bathroom during a meeting at work), our laboratories and classrooms are structured with the implicit assumption that what is on the child's mind mirrors what the adult has in mind. Because children are both less likely to deliberately compartmentalize their experience than adults, and less forceful or clear about how they are interpreting a situation, the distance between their inner life and the outer context has particular ramifications. For example, any assessment of Ben's language comprehension, his ability to plan his actions, or his representation of the conversation or the activities to come would be inadequate without some understanding of what was salient at that moment to him.

THINKING ABOUT WHAT CHILDREN THINK ABOUT

A teacher wrote the following to me:

> The whole class went outside to try to find Olivia's lost gold rabbit pendant, which had been on a chain around her neck. The kids were outside under the picnic table searching when Nicholas shouted, "I just remembered that I saw the gold rabbit here under the picnic table. That means that we have to go and talk to all the classes and find out who took it." It was absolutely untrue because Olivia had just lost it minutes before. Nicholas had the whole class in an uproar. When I said that Nicholas was making it up (because he seems to be doing a lot of that lately), he adamantly refused to acknowledge that he was making it up.
>
> As I thought of the whole incident later, I thought that it was possible that Nicholas might have mixed the incident with a movie or TV show; or his imagination conjured up the whole thing and he was having trouble separating it from reality. Perhaps, on the other hand, he wanted to make this whole event into an adventure and just was enjoying the attention.[33]

This teacher seems to be trying to understand that Nicholas's motivations are different than hers (or Olivia's). But she has jumped to the conclusion that he has lied before fully visualizing the meaning of the episode from his perspective. What did he hear when Olivia announced that she had lost her gold necklace? He heard the tone, and recognized the excitement in her expression. This little boy probably felt excited too, searching around under the picnic table. Much as Jerome Bruner suggests in *Making Stories,* the search may have triggered a story outline in Nicholas's mind, one in which investigation is called for.[34] In fact, that story line was probably much more important to Nicholas than either finding the necklace or telling the truth.

Can research help us figure out what this moment was like from Nicholas's perspective? Yes and no. We can draw on research about children's memory, communication skills, and social relations to understand better why Nicholas would be emphatic about recalling something that could not have happened. He is five, and not likely to work hard to recall where and when he last saw Olivia's necklace. He is also unlikely to think carefully about what his teacher knows or has seen that makes her insist he is making his story up. He seems unperturbed, in fact, that she contradicts his pronouncement. Why? This is where research could be more helpful than it has been so far. What is salient to Nicholas about this situation is quite different than what might be salient to his teacher, or to Olivia. If one were to adopt Nicholas's point of view, certain events and details would be more salient than others. One part of the event would become the "figure," or the most central aspect, and the rest would become the "ground," or backdrop (in the Gestalt sense of "figure" and "ground," in which these aspects can change). From Nicholas's perspective, the episode contains friends and teachers and a lost object inviting drama, with him featured as the hero. Understanding what the experience means to Nicholas is crucial to understanding why he does what he does in that setting.

Figuring out what dots a child is connecting can't always be done based on isolated instances, or on what a child says in one given situation. The dots need to cross time and situation, and need to take unconscious as well as conscious behavior into account. Fortunately, we are not confined to anecdotes, and armchair interpretations of them, for insight into children's experience of themselves in the world. There is a wide range of studies that offer material and information for those of us trying to build a first-person account of early childhood. One can use these to begin to develop a picture of the child's experience, and thus of her inner life.

INCLUDING THE CHILD'S PERSPECTIVE

Besides asking children what they feel and think, what else can we do to get some sense of how the world looks and feels to them? Part of the answer lies in interpreting and using data in a somewhat different way than we have in the past. For example, in a fine study, Paul Harris and Robert Kavanaugh sought to find out just what children thought about the status of a pretend fox hiding in a box. Two children somewhere between the ages of three and five were brought into a lab play room, which contained some furniture and a big cardboard box set against a wall. The experimenter told the children they were going to hear a fun make-believe story about a fox hiding in the box. They were reminded several times that all of this was just make-believe, and then engaged in an exciting story all about whether the fox would be hungry and come out looking for food. At some point the experimenter would say that she forgot something in another room and would be back in a few moments. She left the children alone in the room with the box (and a video camera recording everything from behind a one-way mirror). Kavanaugh and Harris were interested in two aspects of the children's behavior: First, did the children get scared, and somehow begin to believe that a real fox was in the box? And second, in what ways did the children's interaction support or change their construction of the imaginary scenario? They found that children were much more likely to peek into the box if they thought a scary fox was in there than if they thought the fox was not scary. They also found that children supported one another's make-believe. But what is most intriguing about the data, from my perspective, is the transitional nature of the children's behavior. One moment they believe there is a fox in there; the next minute, they don't (and vice versa). One child reassures her friend there is only an imaginary friend in there, and moments later looks scared as if she doesn't believe her own reassurances. The study demonstrates some important points about how and when children use others to construct or elaborate make-believe scenarios.[35] It also suggests that the make-believe frame is shaky when children feel frightened (and when the person who created the frame is not around to support it). The emotional significance of the situation plays a crucial role in children's cognitive functioning. What and how they think about the status of the imaginary creature have everything to do with how scared they are.

On the flip side, as Harris points out in his book *The Work of the Imagination,* imaginary scenarios can produce emotion, as much as emotion can produce imaginative work. A look at the tapes shows some of the children waffling between an exciting sense that there is a make-believe fox about which they can pretend together, and a disturbing sense that maybe something will actually pop out of that box and scare them. The results of the study may show that a certain percentage of children believe the fox is real, while most continue to behave as if the fox is imaginary.[36] But the children's facial expressions, gestures, and words while the experimenter is out of the room show that many of them fluctuate. At one point they seem quite confident that there is no real fox in the box. At another moment they seem frightened (for instance, one little girl leans over and whispers to her friend, "I know in my heart there isn't a fox in there"). This suggests that the usual empirical sieve is not fine enough to catch the vital particles. Changes in the child's experience or behavior over time are well worth tracking.

The fox in the box is a good example of a study that offers at least two levels of insight. One level concerns what kinds of reality/fantasy distinctions children can make at a certain age (do they know the fox is just pretend?), and what kinds of social interaction promote, support, or influence this kind of imaginary thinking. But the second level offers us a sense of what the child sees and thinks during such an experience. In this particular study, a grown-up introduces the pretend scenario, which sets it apart from the bulk of naturally occurring play, since in everyday life it is most often the child who initiates pretend scenarios. The data show that children experience this contrived situation as the unfolding of an exciting story that invites pretense. But as is so often the case, the child's sense of engagement and belief fluctuates, as do her emotions (both in intensity and kind). In other words, at one moment she is intrigued that the experimenter has invited her into a story; at another moment she is scared, and likes it; and a moment later she is a bit too scared, comforts herself, and alters the situation by telling her friend that in her heart she knows the fox is not real. Clearly children at this age are extremely responsive to situation—the presence or absence of an adult and the scariness of the scenario. One cannot isolate the child's cognitive abilities from the situation in which she uses them. Moreover, in order to understand that situation, one has to view it from her perspective, imagine her world at the moment she enters that lab room.

There are also some interesting examples of research that does not focus explicitly on children's experience, but lends itself to such insight, if approached in the right way. The first of these involves one of the most powerful models to emerge in the past thirty years in developmental psychology: the idea of the script. Katherine Nelson, its architect, argues that children form scripts for meaningful routines and well-known events that they encounter. These scripts are organized around socially meaningful goals (eating breakfast, going to a birthday party, going to day care, bedtime, and so on), and include people, places, and actions. They allow the child to make sense of everyday experience, and to separate the ordinary from the unusual (I usually eat toast, but sometimes I have a boiled egg; usually Daddy picks me up, but once he forgot). They provide the child with a basis for all kinds of further cognitive work (developing concepts, creating complex linguistic structures, understanding basic principles such as causality, and so forth).

The research done to support this idea has been ingenious and elegant. For instance, as described in Chapter 2, early research showed that though a child may not be able to tell you how he got ready for bed that evening, he can tell you how he usually gets ready for bed (he may not have a specific representation or memory of last night's activities, but he can describe his mental script for the usual routine). This groundbreaking research rested on a simple modification of an existing research technique. Instead of asking a child "What did you do before bed last night?" you ask, "How do you get ready for bed?" It is worth noting, too, that many of the early descriptions that supported Nelson's theory came from observations of children in everyday situations (talking to one another while playing in day care), in which children discussed and exchanged the scripts they were using.[37]

Later research showed that those early scripts not only help children make sense of their day, but form the basis of more abstract and logical thinking skills. Studies showed that children are more able to answer questions about concepts and categories when they have learned those categories through the enactment of events and scenarios. So for instance, children who are asked to explain the conceptual relationship of lions and tigers to circus animals after encountering toys that make up a circus scenario appear more competent than children who are asked about daisies, roses, and flowers after simply seeing various arrays of these objects. These kinds of studies show how powerful scripts are as a framework for organizing knowledge and action. It is an appealing theory, as well, because it implies that the child's thinking develops in tune with the kinds of events that are meaningful in her community, and it shows that at the most basic level, the child organizes thought around experiences that are socially mediated. But what does this research tell us about the child's experience?

If we imagine the child actively constructing scripts, rearranging them, exploring their limits and their fit with the world, it gives us a wonderful picture of a child venturing forth, continually comparing her expectations about what will happen with what seems to be really happening. The script theory was developed to offer a more realistic and generative account of how the child organizes and represents experience. The theory explained the data well, and it predicted various aspects of what children can and cannot do in various situations. It also gave the child more credit than earlier theories, and it placed more emphasis on a real child making sense of real experience. But it also offers researchers the chance, not yet taken, to imagine in more concrete and precise detail the way a child might think and respond as he encounters expected and unexpected moments in the day.

Let me give another example of research that holds two levels of meaning. We now know that children experience an early set of emotions that are considered primary, and a more mature set of emotions we term secondary. The real difference between these two types of emotion is that the first is fairly direct and primitive (feeling cared for, feeling distress, and so on). The second type is self-conscious. That is, secondary emotions require some awareness of self-in-the-world. Feelings such as pride, for example, require a child to have a sense of who she is, in order to feel satisfaction at her own accomplishments, as well as an awareness of how she seems in the eyes of others. Indeed, such awareness is the beginning of the many selves that James discussed in his chapter on the self: "Properly speaking I have as many selves as there are representations of me in the eyes of others."[38] What is interesting about the work that has led to a distinction between direct emotion and self-conscious emotion is that it helps explain the difference between the child who cries in distress when her mother walks out of the room and the child who cries in shame when he is being teased.[39] But such research also considers distinctions that may feel meaningful or real to the child herself. It allows one to understand behavioral differences that go hand-in-hand with experiential differences.

Take, for example, a three-year-old boy who builds a tall tower of blocks that gets knocked down. He cries in frustration and rage. One can ask a set of behavioral questions about this. Is he able to limit his frustration, refocus, and start building again, or does he become so distracted by his emotions that he dissolves and cannot resume playing? Do words (a suggestion from someone else, or a reprimand) help him get back on track? But one can also explore his experience of this frustration. What story is he telling himself about what is happening? Is there an important difference between the child too young to tell such a story to herself, and the one who experiences such frustration in a more mediated, self-conscious way?

Jerome Kagan's seminal work on temperament offers another view. Kagan has shown, quite convincingly, that children as young as four months, and probably younger, exhibit signs of distinctive temperaments. Specifically, Kagan has shown that you can tell from watching a four-month-old respond to something like a new mobile whether the baby is inhibited or uninhibited. Babies who get easily distressed by new stimuli, and further distressed by their own heightened response, are likely to be timid later in life. Babies who react with a momentary pause or heightened interest, but take it in stride and quickly go back to their usual level of activity (making sounds, kicking their feet, looking around) are likely to be uninhibited later in life (respond easily to new situations). These data have been used to trace the stability of temperament and to identify causes of instability.[40] What has been less examined using these data is how temperament might shape a child's response to a vast array of experiences. The shy or inhibited child is going to construe the world quite differently than the uninhibited child. Dennie Wolf and her colleagues have found, for instance, that shy children tell fewer stories of personal experience to their peers than children who are not shy.[41] Imagine the shy child who experiences an accelerated heartbeat, flushed skin, and a sense of apprehension as she enters a room full of peers. Contrast this with the child who sees the room as a beehive of invitations and opportunities to play and interact with friends and foes. Now imagine that the child who is not shy is sitting down at the drawing table, busily boasting to his friends about the new car his father got. The shy child, meanwhile, is not telling any stories about herself, nor seeing her reflection through the responses of her audience. Kagan's temperament research, when thought through in context and in terms of the child's experience of daily situations, takes on a whole new level of meaning beyond the profound one it has already offered us. Topics such as temperament and emotion need to be looked at not only as causes of behavior, but also as kinds of experience that may explain certain developmental changes.

One of the most interesting things we have learned since Piaget concerns the general versus specific nature of how children develop knowledge and cognitive skills. We all know that children seem to get better at a vast array of things as they age, and that they seem to know more. Piaget gave us the groundbreaking view that there are across-the-board, pervasive shifts, revolutions really, in the way the child's mind takes in and organizes knowledge. This formulation helps us understand why you can talk until you are blue in the face to a two-year-old about why 2 + 5 is the same as 5 + 2 and your words will literally have no meaning for her, whereas a seven-year-old may well find this to be an intriguing and eventually sensible conversation. I mentioned earlier that a growing number of researchers have found evidence for the idea that knowledge, and sophistication in thinking, develops locally—that is, in one domain at a time. Micheline Chi found that children who were chess experts had much more sophisticated ways of remembering positions of chess pieces than nonexpert chess players.[42] But those same children were not necessarily better at remembering in other settings, where other kinds of memory skills are involved. Contrary to Piaget's claims, Chi found that memory functions differently within a person's area of expertise than elsewhere. One's memory is not a general skill applied to all domains, but functions at different levels and in different ways depending on the individual's previous experience and skill within the domain. This means that not all four-year-olds are alike, and that what a four-year-old has been doing (what objects she is exposed to, what activities she spends her time on, what kinds of knowledge she has amassed, what is demanded of her in daily life) will have a strong influence on the kind and level of her cognitive skills. Being an expert or a novice at something turns out to be as relevant as one's age. The methodological implications of this finding are important. A child's specific experiences must be taken into account when characterizing her cognitive abilities, and we must be careful about generalizing from one experimental setting to another.

More recently, research conducted by Susan Carey has shown that while there are certain general principles or skills that all young children may use to make their way into a new domain, once there they need specific encounters with the materials and processes of that domain to become more skilled and therefore more developed in their thinking about that domain. Carey and her colleagues called the initial, launching skills "skeletal principles"—they guide the child's attention, and provide them with certain basic ways of organizing and remembering information or procedures.[43] But beyond that, the ways of thinking and operating can only be gleaned from interactions with the materials or tasks involved. For instance, in one study Chi has compared children who know a lot about dinosaurs to children who don't. Young dinosaur experts show a more sophisticated and powerful set of reasoning skills when asked to solve problems involving those dinosaurs than children of the same age who do not know a lot about dinosaurs.

This kind of research invites another equally important kind of investigation, one that seeks to put together a picture of how the world looks to these young experts and nonexperts. Imagine for a moment two children walking into a room that contains a wide assortment of toy dinosaurs (or any other collection of objects associated with a discipline, a domain, or a kind of work). One child immediately feels comfortable, seeing familiar objects. The objects fall quickly and easily into useful groups of some sort, and some mental or physical activity beckons the child (I can sort these, I can create my favorite Jurassic Park game with these, I can peel these and eat them, I can use these to build something, and so forth). The other child may be fascinated and drawn into the room. But she may instead spend time looking at the objects, wondering what they are. She may be drawn to one in particular, without an overarching sense of how they all go together. She may be uncertain how to use the objects, and her attention to details such as color, shape, names, or functions may shift. In other words, expertise changes the quality of a child's experience.

A MORE COMPLETE VIEW OF CHILDHOOD

When Piaget sat down to watch his children, Jacqueline, Lucienne, and Laurent, what kind of child did he see? A child playing with objects. This child was, he claimed, discovering principles of how the world worked. Her mind incorporated new experiences into old expectations (what he called schemas), and she used this process of revision as a way of expanding her understanding of the world. Piagetians since then, and even those who have presented themselves as critics of Piaget, have led us to imagine a child much like a scientist—one who revises theory to account for new data. Piaget saw what Paul Harris has termed a stubborn autodidact: a child resolutely teaching herself knowledge and skills through trial and error with the physical world, limited only by her own internal level of development (her schemas). This child did not seem all that attuned to the feelings, values, and thoughts of those around her. Nor did the knowledge she acquired bear the mark of others—that is, her knowledge was not what some might term local, but rather was based on universal principles. Since Piaget, some have worked to expand and refine his theory, while others have offered strong alternatives to it. But somehow all have spoken to it, one way or another.

What do I see when I look at a three- or four-year-old playing? I too see a child who is drawn into experimenting with the world around her. But this child, and her explorations, are more sensual, more attuned to aesthetics, and more reflective than most developmental research would lead one to believe. The tremendous focus on cognitive processes, and our accumulation of evidence regarding the impressive problem-solving skills of young children, have drawn our attention away from other aspects of the intellectual life of the young child—her musings about the meaning of events, her reflections on possible interpretations of things, and her curiosity about representations themselves. Though research over the past fifty years has refined and even in some cases refuted Piaget's conclusions, the child depicted by most research is still highly rational, goal-oriented, and sensible. Ironically Piaget himself often described a child thinking about his or her world in a probing, reflective way, but this strand of his work was not amplified in much of the work that followed.

Meanwhile, researchers have certainly discovered that the very young child (eighteen months to four years) is more attuned to the social world than Piaget thought, and many have demonstrated the ways in which the child eagerly and intuitively seeks to learn the rules and codes of her culture. When I close my eyes and imagine a four-year-old drawn from my years of observation, I don't see a child alone with pebbles but rather a child in a room with other people—parents, caregivers, siblings, and peers. The child may or may not be acting in a solitary way, but those people, her image and awareness of them, and their influence on her behavior, are central to understanding how and what she thinks. She is looking at the pebbles, and then looking to see if her mother is too. She hands a pebble to the other child and waits to see what he will do with it. She makes a pattern with the pebbles, and gauges the teacher's facial response as she thinks about how to rearrange the pattern. The teacher suggests another way of placing the pebbles, which the little girl tries. This leads her to realize that the pebbles can be arranged to create a symbol, and thereby represent something else. Research over the past sixty years on the role of other people in the child's development of knowledge allows us to imagine a child who experiences the physical world, and develops her knowledge of such a world, through her experiences with others.

One important change in how we view children is that we now see them as budding experts who absorb information and ideas from experts within their culture, and who practice, amassing strategies, information, and techniques that lift their thinking to a higher level within that domain or discipline. Their knowledge therefore is both culturally specific and domain specific. Children's skills emerge from experience with a certain set of materials and goals, and reflect the community and habits within which they are learned and used.

By emphasizing action as a way of knowing, Piaget somehow led us to a child who rarely ruminates, fantasizes, or reflects on her own thoughts, actions, or interactions. But knowing how you know, knowing that others know something different from you, and thinking about your own knowledge are essential aspects of becoming a mature problem solver. This sense of a child developing his own consciousness in relation to the consciousness of others has been missing from our collective image of children, even while the research has shown increasingly that metacognition is a key to acquiring cognitive strategies and skills.

We have to be careful, however, not to require too much self-awareness or metacognition from the young child. For instance, a child may pretend, and understand that others are pretending, without any explicit theory or explanation for what this means. While children probably have rich, lively, and complex inner thoughts about what they are doing and experiencing, this does not mean they are articulating rational explanations in their minds for what is going on. As Angeline Lillard and Katherine Nelson have both pointed out, children need not have theories the way scientists do in order to engage in the explorations and tasks that derive from that theory.[44]

Children often can engage in subtle and complex mental processes (like deciding what is make-believe) without being able to explain to another person why they are doing it, or even that they are doing it. And that brings us to the understanding that was implicit even in Piaget's work, but never sufficiently developed: What guides and explains the child's experience (as well as much of her behavior) is neither comfort, pleasure, nor cognitive understanding. Instead she is busily constructing meaning about her body, her thoughts, the people around her, and the physical world. This search for meaning unifies the different ways in which she functions, and helps us understand not only her strategies and behaviors, but also her experience of everyday life. But this is never a dry investigation of a static and cool physical world. It is a juicy investigation, replete with moments of tension, pleasure, fantasy, and triumph. These hotter feelings do not merely accompany the child's emerging knowledge but shape it. The child is continually constructing stories, images, plans, and explanations that make her experiences and encounters meaningful to her. That is, her stories and explanations reveal, as well as inform, her interpretations of experience. Further, these interpretations are as important as any behavior or ability she exhibits in an experimental setting.

Recently I visited a kindergarten classroom containing twenty-one children ranging in age from four to six-and-a-half (an unusually wide range for a conventional public school). After a short meeting in which the teacher went over a morning message and discussed the schedule for the day, the children dispersed to various work and play areas. Two little girls headed straight for the dollhouse area, where they began to enact a tea scene, including two small stuffed animals belonging to one of the girls, Kayla, who is just under five-and-a-half years old. They were very happy and congenial in their play, and even happy to accept a little boy who had been lingering watchfully on the outskirts of the doll area until the teacher suggested, "Here Scott, why don't you join them. They're playing . . . well, why don't they tell you what they're playing. Kayla, Scott is going to join you." Kayla responded happily, "Okay. We're playing house." Scott sat down at the table, and they continued drinking their tea (lifting small plastic cups to their mouths). At some point Kayla said to the other little girl that the dog was upset. He doesn't like it when people he doesn't know are around (perhaps referring to me—I am sitting on a small chair just outside the play area). Later she said to her friend, "What am I gonna do, Mom? My doggy's sick." The other little girl suggested, "Put him in the hat" (a black cowboy hat that is hanging upside down from a hook, serving as a hammock, as well as a hospital of some sort, for two other small stuffed animals). As Kayla put her dog in the hat, the little boy Scott got down on all fours and began to meow. Kayla said, somewhat severely and with a frown, "You're not a cat." He paused, uncertain, in his meowing, but didn't get off the floor. The second little girl said, "Well, he's PLAYING cat." Okay, Kayla said, and he continued meowing while they drank tea and discussed the health of the animals in the hat. Finally the teacher rang a bell and announced that it was time to clean up and get ready for the work time. Kayla began to sob. The assistant went over to her to find out why she was so upset. Crying loudly, and clinging to the puppy dog and a small stuffed cat, she said, "I don't WANT to put my dog and cat away for work time. I want to keep them." The teacher explained that the children cannot have toys during work time. "But I want them to watch me doing math." The teacher agreed to place the small animals on a ledge near the rug where the children gather to discuss work time and get their instructions and folders from the teacher. When it was time to get up and get her folder and walk over to a table, Kayla again became distressed, saying to the teacher, "They can't see me when I'm sitting over here. Where can I put them so that they can watch me do my math?" The most striking thing about this scenario is that the little girl can think quickly and flexibly about the difference between what she can see and what the dog and cat can see from various positions in the room (it is the three-mountain task in real life). But this cognitive sophistication is made manifest through her intense worry about what a stuffed animal can see.

The child I see vacillates more dramatically between modes of thought and is more imaginative and actively engaged in construing her world than Piaget and many researchers since then would lead us to envision. But the account offered here is just a beginning. More descriptive research is needed to characterize development as it really happens. Such research would dramatically benefit the work of both teachers and researchers.

5

Why This Matters, and to Whom

In 2000, the *Onion* published a small humorous piece in which the author described something called Youthful Tendency Disorder:

> Day after day, upon arriving home from pre-school, Caitlin would retreat into a bizarre fantasy world. Sometimes she would pretend to be people and things she was not. Other times, without warning, she would burst into nonsensical song. Some days she would run directionless through the backyard of the Sernas' comfortable Redlands home, laughing and shrieking as she chased imaginary objects.
>
> When months of sessions with a local psychologist failed to yield an answer, Nicholas and Beverly took Caitlin to a prominent Los Angeles pediatric neurologist for more exhaustive testing. Finally, on Sept. 11, the Sernas received the heartbreaking news: Caitlin was among a growing legion of U.S. children suffering from Youthful Tendency Disorder.[1]

The author's point, hilariously conveyed, is that many adults seem to find the behaviors and moods so essential to the nature of childhood to be a problem in a world where we increasingly want children to straighten up, learn what they need to learn, and get ready for the world of work. Though the author may have hoped that his spoof seemed outrageous, the view he satirizes is all too familiar. Many of our daily expectations regarding our children (whether they are actually our offspring, or our students) suggest that we have a distorted view of childhood. Too many of our practices (as parents and teachers) rest on misguided assumptions about children and the nature of development. In some cases, these practices reflect a lack of knowledge about child development. More disturbing is the possibility that current research in developmental psychology itself often leads to some of these inappropriate expectations and practices.

One April, while visiting my parents in eastern Long Island, I took my eight-year-old son to walk on the beach. A woman about my age was lying in the sand, watching as two girls, about nine years old, played and talked nearby. It was about 3:30 in the afternoon, and I realized that she had brought her daughter and her daughter's friend to play on the beach after school. Soon after I noticed them, the daughter teased the other girl about something. The mother called out in a disapproving voice, reminding her not to tease her friend. A few minutes later the teasing had escalated into bickering, though it was not at all clear to an outsider that either girl was unhappy. The mother called her daughter over in an aggravated tone and said, reproachfully, "Trudy, now is this what you would call a successful play date?" The girl looked down, briefly daunted, said nothing, and returned to her friend. This might seem funny if it weren't so depressing to hear a parent characterize two children's time together as a successful (or by implication, unsuccessful) play date. Even the term play date implies that play occurs as a circumscribed and planned activity, rather than an activity and orientation that pervade the child's day. It implies that when there is no play date, other things must be happening: work, learning, and so forth. One could argue that this distinction merely reflects the culture in which we live—a culture that draws a thick boundary between work and play. But a sharp distinction between work and play is antithetical to the way young children (even children as old as nine), experience the world and therefore goes against the grain of development. Moreover, the idea of a successful play date is downright grim. One wonders what will mark it as a success or a failure among children who have the normal array of social skills and concerns. Though just an anecdote, the "successful" play-date story illustrates, first, how even the most offhand comments and gestures rest on and/or reflect underlying perspectives on childhood, and second, the current, misguided view adults in our culture have of children. Such offhand comments and gestures can interfere with children's understanding of their own development—their perception of what is normal and okay. Moreover, this view focuses attention on success and failure, and leads us to look for signs that the child is edging closer to what she should and could become. The child is seen almost completely in terms of how close she is to approximating adult abilities.

But if parents harbor such developmentally off-base views, current research is partly to blame. Such research has both rested on and perpetuated a view of children as incomplete adults, and led to a distorted concept of children. In addition, this way of thinking about development has helped to create a constricting and unproductive atmosphere for real children in real situations, such as school.

A sobering example of this shift was the announcement in Chicago several years ago that recess would be shortened to give more learning time to elementary school students. Several other states and school districts have made similar changes. This change is a direct result of thinking that young children could learn more (become more adultlike faster) if they just spent more time doing the desired activity or skill. It also reflects a belief that play is not important to children. Completely absent from this decision was any understanding of the true nature of developmental progress, or the psychological characteristics of young children. This is very discouraging. It means that though we have learned a lot in recent years about the differences between young children and older children or grown-ups, we have, if anything, slipped backward in our understanding of what they should and can be doing during those early years to optimize not only their experience in the moment, but also their development. Though we have long since understood that children are qualitatively different from adults, we continue, much of the time, to treat them like small adults.

THE FALLACY OF THE STRAIGHT PATH TO LEARNING

I have asked over one hundred teachers and parents why they believe elementary-school-aged children should have homework. Invariably their answer is that later on children will have to do homework (when they are in middle and high school) and that they might as well get into the habit of it. In other words, homework at age six prepares the child for homework at age sixteen. This commonly used logic offers an example of the implicit and often unexamined assumptions people use when thinking about children's development. Most people in our culture have some inchoate idea about which processes in development are continuous and stable (doing a little homework at age six will somehow lead to doing even better homework at age sixteen) and which processes are less obvious or linear. For example, if you ask most parents in the United States about when their children should begin to have sexual intercourse, few would suggest that they should begin by age six so that they will be good at it by the time they are age twenty-one. Most parents, even if they don't know it, assume that some processes are accumulative and others are more indirect, involving qualitative leaps and changes.

But if there is one thing developmental research has shown, it is that the experiences and processes that lead to a given skill or ability do not necessarily look like that skill or ability in its full-blown form. Take, for example, early signs of conversational ability and the mature ability to engage in dialogue. Few watching a baby waiting expectantly to be tickled, laughing when tickled, and then waiting to be tickled again would jump to thoughts of conversations. Yet it is just that kind of reciprocity in infancy that psychologists believe is a precursor to the back and forth of conversations in childhood and adulthood. Developmental psychologists often try to identify the precursors and prerequisites of important abilities. In many cases, experiences and processes that are developmentally connected do not appear to be. For example, it is very common for parents (and many classroom teachers) to treat learning the alphabet as the first and perhaps essential step in learning to read. But research by Gordon Wells in Bristol, England, in which he fitted two- and three-year-olds with small vests that had microphones attached to them, revealed, among other things, that children who engaged in more conversations at home as toddlers learned to read more easily and sooner than children who came from families in which there were fewer and briefer conversations between adults and children.[2] This illustrates the central developmental tenet that a given experience at time A may be essential for, and lead to, a certain ability or experience at time B, but that superficially these two processes or activities might look nothing alike (for example, casual conversations with parents lead to reading skills in school). For those adults who raise and educate children, the implications of this finding are huge. Instead of believing that every desired trait, habit, and ability must be inculcated early on, one begins to look for experiences that will lead to the desired ability, however indirectly. A thoughtful look at how teachers are teaching shows that this subtle but pervasive principle of development is rarely evident in classrooms today.

My favorite example of the disconnect between how children truly learn and how they are taught was told to me by a parent and involves an eight-year-old student in a suburban elementary school and her third-grade teacher. The little girl, Ruth, had told a long story at the dinner table about a squirrel family. Her father suggested that she use the story the next time she was asked to write in class. "Oh, I can't do that," Ruth said. "We can only write about things that have really happened to us." Though surprised by this, the father said nothing. A few days later he called his daughter's teacher. "Yes," the teacher assured him, "we tell them that. We find that when they make up stories, they get lost in the process. Their stories are much clearer and better if we hold them to the facts." What a startling thing to hear from someone who supposedly knows about children. It seems that the teachers in this particular school had held a long series of meetings to talk about how to improve their writing program. They had decided to focus the children on personal narratives, with the idea that real experience provides children with a natural and readily available organizational structure for their stories. They felt that the narratives would be more clearly written if the children were told to not make anything up, or mix facts with fiction. The teacher told Ruth's father that in her experience, when children begin to add made-up elements to the story, they become absorbed in the act of storytelling and lose sight of the final product. What strikes me about this example is the way in which good research on children's personal narratives has been filtered down and (mis)used in the classroom.

The teacher's original goal is an important and good one—to find ways to help children write well. The teachers want elementary-school-aged children to understand how to include a beginning, middle, and an end in their story. Understandably, they want children to learn how to keep to the plot, how to flesh out their characters, how to focus on one problem or high point, and how to clearly convey a story. Their sense that personal experiences will provide children with rich topics for writing makes sense as well. But the teacher's concern that mixing facts and fiction will muddy the writing, and that children should not get "lost in the process," reflects a misunderstanding of the developmental process.

Implicit in this particular educational practice is the idea that children should do at age eight what we want them to do at forty years old (write clearly, with an audience in mind, aware all the time of the finished product). Nowhere in that teacher's educational plan is an acknowledgment that eight-year-olds may need to use stories in ways different than those used by adults, but ways that may be precursors, or even prerequisites, of adult skills. Based on some research, a teacher might well take the view that getting lost in the process of storytelling when you are eight is exactly what leads to clarity and audience awareness at forty. An eight-year-old may not use stories to communicate as much as she uses them to think out loud. It is entirely plausible that in order to be a good adult writer, you have to have plenty of experience getting "lost in the story" when you are young.

Such a view is not particularly radical. Those who subscribe to the idea that a solid early attachment between mother and toddler leads to greater security and comfort with separation for the preschooler understand that just because you do a lot of something when you are little, like clinging to your mother, does not mean you will need to go on doing it into adulthood. Quite the contrary, the more you get of what you need as a toddler, the less you need it later.

The anecdote about Ruth's writing experience suggests that teaching practices fail to reflect a deep understanding of development in two ways. First, often teachers and parents do not seem to understand the nature of psychological development. Though not the focus of this book, this is a serious problem: developmental psychologists have not done a good enough job talking about their findings to parents and those who work with children in a manner that is both approachable and richly informative. It is also the case that schools don't often demand that the teachers they hire have more than a cursory knowledge of the most superficial aspects of child and adolescent development.

The second layer to the problem rests with the research itself. As mentioned earlier, research on psychological development describes a child whose development is linear, and whose mind is rational, orderly, and task oriented. People readily accept and use such a model of the child, even though a few days of careful observation in a day care center prove it wrong. That is not to say that the studies themselves are inaccurate or poorly done, but that taken together they lead to an inadequate view of the child's inner life. Whether a teacher or a researcher, if you are looking only for signs of pre-adult behavior, or hints of a budding logician, that is likely to be all you will find. If, however, you have your eyes open for signs that children are making sense of their world, you will be much more likely to identify moments in which the children are shifting between frames of reference and ways of constructing reality.

DEVELOPMENTAL PSYCHOLOGY MATTERS

Toward the end of her classic book *Children's Minds,* published in 1978, Margaret Donaldson explains that by the time they come to school, all normal children can show skill as thinkers and language users, so long as they are dealing with "real-life," meaningful situations in which they participate with their own purposes and intentions and in which they can recognize and respond to purposes and intentions in others. Her argument is deceptively simple—we cannot fully appreciate or nurture the young child's mental development until we recognize how important it is for him to make sense of whatever task he must do, or skill he must learn.[3]

But in order to understand the child's mind, and to present the child with tasks that are meaningful to her, we need to have a sufficiently rich and dynamic view of what the child's inner life is like. Almost a decade after Donaldson wrote *Children's Minds,* Jerome Bruner picked up her theme and took it further. At the end of his book *Actual Minds, Possible Worlds,* he argues that the stakes of this challenge are high indeed, and that the multidimensional way that children approach the world demands to be understood.

> When and if we pass beyond the unspoken despair in which we are now living, when we feel we are again able to control the race to destruction, a new breed of developmental theory is likely to arise. It will be motivated by the question of how to create a new generation that can prevent the world from dissolving into chaos and destroying itself. I think that its central technical concern will be how to create in the mind of the young an appreciation of the fact that many worlds are possible, that meaning and reality are created and not discovered, that negotiation is the art of constructing new meanings by which individuals can regulate their relations with each other.[4]

Donaldson and Bruner notwithstanding, mainstream developmental psychology has failed to take into account children's powerful need to make sense of themselves and their worlds. Children's drive (and ability) to make sense is key to their cognitive work. But when we place children in situations that don't make sense to them, we cannot see what they are really like. Our failure to recognize their need to make sense and their proclivity to interpret what is happening to them limits what we can know about them. Whether we can see it or not, children are always in the process of constructing explanations, sequences, predictions, and stories that render the world meaningful to them. The key word in Bruner's passage is "meaning," because it is meaning, rather than logic, that drives the child's thoughts and helps explain her actions. Children in their daily lives, asking questions, making things up, enacting scenarios, and solving problems, show to the careful observer their relentless and often exuberant effort to construct meaning. I use the word meaning here to refer to the interpretations children use to make sense of their experience—the meaning of an event, action, or occurrence usually includes the child's sense of how that event or action fits into his world, who is doing what and for what purpose, and how words, looks, and gestures within that event or action should be construed. I am not offering a strict or experimental definition here, but rather suggesting that children are constantly making sense of what goes on around them. What is "sensible" to a three-year-old, however, might not be the same as what is "sensible" to a scientist, or any other adult. The young child's meanings may or may not fit an adult pattern, and may or may not lead to short-term solutions for the child, but they do offer us a view of their inner lives and thus may provide long-term approaches to guiding children as they develop.

Teachers, parents, and researchers influence one another in several ways. Prevailing cultural values and habits influence the researcher's focus. But parents and teachers, in turn, are influenced by experiments and scientific claims about young children. For instance, in a culture that values test-taking skills and sees high test scores as a measure of someone's ability, parents and teachers will focus on optimizing their children's test-taking abilities. Similarly, researchers will try to find out more about the causes of low test scores, and the long-term consequences of low test scores in childhood. But often the mutual influence of teachers, parents, and researchers plays itself out on a subtler level. These groups of people confirm and support one another's implicit model of what children are like.

Ever since I myself taught young children, I have seen teachers, and sometimes parents, take an angry or out-of-control child gently (or ungently) by the shoulders and tell her to spend a few minutes in a chair, in a quiet space in the room, thinking about what has just happened. This has always seemed ridiculous to me, antithetical to what children are all about. How can a child, at a stage in which she thinks with her body, think about something while sitting down? There are, no doubt, other reasons why this approach works some of the time. It may serve as a negative reinforcement, which discourages or extinguishes the naughty behavior, for a while, in that classroom. Sitting down for five minutes might also simply give a child a chance to change gears, calm down, or rest, any of which might be just the ticket for redirecting her behavior. What it probably will not do, however, is lead to some interesting thinking on the child's part about what she has done or what she is feeling.

What is in the mind of the teacher at the moment he or she suggests that this four-year-old spend a few minutes in "time-out"? The model, implicit or explicit, features a child able to direct her thoughts at will, able to think about feeling and action without acting, and without feeling too much. Such a view, common as it is, just doesn't make sense.

PEEKING INTO THE CHILD'S MIND

One of the teachers I have known for a long time, a warm and skilled, though old-fashioned, kindergarten teacher who has taught for thirty years in a rural one-room schoolhouse, recounted the following story about a favorite student of hers, Milo.

> Recently, a friend of mine spent the morning observing my class. After the morning, my friend asked me who the handsome dark child

> was (it was Milo). She laughed and told me about Milo during story time. I ask all the children to sit on the floor in front of me with their hands clasped in front of them, so that they will learn to sit quietly, and won't fidget. My friend saw that Milo had solemnly kept his hands clasped in his lap whenever I was looking at the group of children seated before me. But every time my head turned down as I focused on the pages in the book, his eyes would open wide, his mouth would spread into a surprised circle, and he would lift up both hands, with fingers spread, in front of him, like two stop signs. The minute I looked back toward the children, his hands would snap together and rest back in his lap, and his face would assume a calm, blank expression.

Whereas a teacher might respond to this news by planning how to get Milo to be less mischievous, or worrying whether his mischief was preventing him from hearing the story and learning the material, there is a more interesting and valuable question: What was that reading period all about for Milo? The answer: Many things all at once. Several strands of impulse, ability, and focus are in play at any given time in a given child's life experience. For Milo, at age five, the interest of challenging the teacher's rule (of clasped hands), of playing with the possibility of getting caught, and of hearing a story are interwoven. Within his mind, there was a shifting balance between two kinds of "here and now"—the here and now of the story, and the here and now of the story-listening situation. The teacher who told me this anecdote clearly appreciated how Milo experienced the moment, and this appreciation shaped the way she worked with Milo in her classroom. In the spirit of her sensitivity to Milo's experience, the dynamic, contextualized, and phenomenological view of children proposed in this book has some very specific implications for those who live and work with children.

The Vital Importance of Play

Play is a central and vital process during childhood. It is not merely that children need time to unwind or have fun. Rather, without play they will be much less likely to develop just the kinds of thinking we feel are so vital to a productive and intelligent adult life. Recent research has shown that not all cultures encourage play in childhood, and clearly children in those cultures grow up to be productive, well-adjusted members of their community. I make no claims here about those communities. My arguments focus on children in my culture, and on the kinds of skills and orientations we seem to value. Just as more and more schools take away play time to make more time for studying, test preparation, and the absorption of new facts, research is making it ever more clear that in order to develop complex mental abilities, children must have plenty of opportunity to construct spheres of reality, transform familiar objects and gestures, create scenarios, and discover the principles that underlie the social and physical worlds in which they live.

Perhaps if teachers understood in a more richly informed and concrete way just what it is children learn and acquire through their play, they would be more likely to give it more attention, time, and space within their classrooms. Play is not a way of making hard work seem attractive (turning a lesson into a "game"), nor is it a time-out from real learning. Instead, when children are given plenty of time and encouragement for their play, they initiate and sustain complex scenarios, experiments, and inquiries in the pursuit of skills, without any direct instruction. Many of the kinds of thinking our culture most values in older children and adults have their roots in the kinds of spontaneous play in which children engage, when given half a chance. There have been brief periods when psychologists have successfully convinced parents and teachers that they should encourage young children to play, and that by doing so, children would develop skills and abilities that would be valuable later in life. In recent years, however, attention has shifted away from the intrinsic value of play as a vital process in development. Those researchers who have focused on play have emphasized how play allows scientific or rational forms of thought to develop. They have seen play as a type of activity, or as a context for examining underlying thought processes, but too few psychologists have focused on playfulness, and the kinds of thinking and navigating the world inherent in play, as essential components of child development.

The Fully Engaged Child

It is clear if you watch children closely that most of them are physically active as they move in and out of play and switch among the various domains outlined in Chapter 3. Piaget argued that the earliest form of knowing is through action.[5] He was interested in the ways in which children's actions are a first kind of representation. But an implication of this view is that children must use their bodies to think. The importance of the mobile body does not end once a child develops mental representation, and can therefore think about something (balance, order, the relationship between objects) without actually touching it. Piaget said that to silence the tongue was to silence the mind. His research goes further than this, however, and implies that to silence the body is to still the mind. Over and over again, in my own observations of children, as well as my readings of my colleagues' research, I see how deeply embodied a child's thinking is, and how hard it is to get a three-dimensional view of her cognitive processes if she isn't doing what she does in everyday life—bouncing, bending, hopping, blowing up her cheeks, grabbing, and flopping down on the ground. In Chapter 3, I described an essay by Claudia Lewis in which she recounts a young boy's use of his body as he tells his peers the sound a dinosaur makes. Given this view of the young child, it is hard to imagine valuable learning taking place without the freedom to move about. But a child's need to use his body can pose a big problem for a teacher of twenty children. That many children using their bodies to explore their thoughts and impressions could create an awfully noisy and wild classroom. Yet even if teachers need to make concessions to orderliness and quiet, it seems imperative to find ways not only to tolerate but also to encourage children to use their bodies, to move around and touch things as they think. It would be a great mistake to assume that this kind of freedom is only important in nursery school. In fact there is a growing body of research suggesting that many kinds of thought are accompanied or facilitated by various types of sensation and movement. We don't yet know just how old one has to be to solve problems, think, imagine, speculate, and weigh alternatives without moving. The best rule, until good research tells us otherwise, is to let children use their bodies as long as it seems intrinsic to their mental activity. The impulse in educational settings is often to insist on the behavior that we expect children to attain eventually (such as sitting still while you learn), instead of allowing behaviors that seem characteristic of the child's current stage. People need to focus on the present state of the child, rather than the imagined future state. The teacher has to be willing to pay close attention to his students to see if they still need room and opportunity to move about as they think, and he should accommodate that need as much as possible.

The "Inconsistent" Child

Though this book draws on a wide range of research and observation conducted over many years by many impressive researchers, it also relies heavily on my own systematic observations of children both alone and with others, at day care centers and schools. I have tried to model my own observations on those collected by naturalists. I have made careful, detailed descriptions of my young subjects doing what they ordinarily do in their own habitat—in this case, their homes, parks, and day cares or schools. As many have noted, the disadvantage of this approach is that one cannot isolate variables that explain behavior, and one cannot test predictions or hypotheses. The great value of this naturalist approach, however, is that it allows a kind of detailed, close picture of what children are like that more controlled experiments often fail to provide. One of the things I have been struck by in my observations is how changeable most children are in everyday life. They are often, in quick succession, happy, then sad, motionless and absorbed by something they are watching, then rushing quickly into an activity that has only just caught their attention. There is a kind of fluctuation to their activity that is the rule rather than the exception. This fluctuation, which may be intrinsic to childhood, appears as inconsistency to a teacher whose mental model of childhood focuses on the future adult. But it is at the least futile, and at the worst, destructive, to try and insist on steadiness and consistency in children. Just because a child flits between several activities, or modes of learning, does not mean he is not seriously engaged, or working on important cognitive problems. It simply means that the young human organism works best by vacillating between different tempos, modes of exploration, media, and foci. So how is the teacher to learn the difference between a productive, engaged child who is simply shifting among spheres, and one who is distracted, restless, disengaged, or disruptive? A child who is engaged and busy, though shifting tempo, focus, and mode of processing, is likely to remain self-directed, even as he moves from one activity to another, or one mindset to another. A child who is restless or disruptive, by contrast, doesn't seem engaged in anything, even for a few moments. Often teachers mistake a child who is resisting the classroom structure or routine for a child who has trouble learning, or has trouble with sustained activity. A child who by six or seven years old cannot do what the teacher asks may continue to have all kinds of difficulties in school. But such resistance does not necessarily mean that the child has trouble becoming engaged in learning, or is incapable of sustained activity. This is yet another argument for giving children more control over their day. The kinds of shifts among domains and spheres of experience that I have observed in my research suggest that when children can make the changes without consequence, they get a lot more out of their activities than when they are devoting a lot of energy to explaining themselves, avoiding constrictions, or trying to comply by resisting these essential shifts altogether.

If this sort of flux is intrinsic to childhood, then teachers should not expect academic progress, understanding, or attention to be steady. I am not recommending that we shorten the time of any given lesson or activity even more (most schools already have periods that are ridiculously short), but instead that we change our conception of what an engaged child looks like and what a student in a classroom should be doing. Children need the opportunity to move, both physically and psychologically.

Recently a friend was considering which of two public-school kindergarten classrooms to request for her five-year-old daughter. She visited each. In one the teacher said that the room was geared toward the "younger" five-year-old, and that she absolutely did not, would not, teach reading. It was, she stressed, a nonacademic kindergarten. Then my friend visited the other kindergarten. This classroom, she was told, was definitely for older five-year-olds. The focus was strongly on academics, and the expectation was that every child would learn to read. I can just imagine the well-intentioned reasoning of the teachers or administrators who set up such an alternative: some kindergarteners are ready to read and others are not. Thus why not create two classrooms, each designed to meet the needs of one group? The biggest problem with this neat, well-defined plan is that children aren't that neat or well-defined as they acquire skills and reconstrue their worlds. Many children are readers one day, block-builders another. The same child who seems completely immersed in a world of dramatic play in September may appear to suddenly launch herself into the world of print in March. But even more likely, the same child who wants to read on Monday morning may need to play in a sandbox on Tuesday and Wednesday.

Why would any classroom arbitrarily separate academics and play, disrupting the possibility of expanding children's experiences and skills with both? What possible good can come of it? Such a strategy seems to have little to do with the way young minds develop.

Instead, the more classrooms can allow for a wide range of types of activities and modes of functioning, the more likely children are to fully exploit their marvelous potential for exploring and developing different types of thinking and modes of reality.

The Value of Interweaving Reality and Fantasy

Observations and experiments show again and again that of the ways in which children shift and vacillate among spheres of experience, one of the most salient and interesting (to them and to us) is that between fantasy and reality. Earlier in this book I argued that an interplay between reality and fantasy is intrinsic to the developmental process and a wonderful, healthy part of growing up. Teachers thus should beware of creating rules and boundaries that preclude such shifting. The story of the teacher insisting that children write stories based only on their real experience violates what we know about how children construct narratives, and what we now know about the value of their playing with the boundaries between types of narratives. Valuing play also means that the kind of playfulness that children often interject into the "serious" business of school is viewed not as a distraction, but a component of good learning for many children. The child who inserts some wishful thinking or exaggeration into their stories and reports may be in fact doing just what he needs to in order to develop a rich understanding of the ways in which the world can be represented. Teachers need to learn better how to capitalize on such playfulness rather than restrict or prohibit it.

IMAGINING THE CHILD'S INNER WORLD

It strikes me as ironic that adults (particularly researchers, but teachers as well) have been so concerned with the child's developing ability to think from another person's point of view when in fact we have so often failed to think carefully and deeply from the child's point of view. For a teacher this one skill is far more powerful than all the facts about developmental psychology that might be learned in a child-development course or textbook. But adopting a child's-eye view requires careful, close observation, and then the time and determination to think about those observations and imagine the mind that accompanied the actions. Researchers and teachers alike need to heed Piaget's most powerful contribution to the scientific study of children's thinking: a recognition that we need to find out more about how they think about the world. The first step of this understanding can often be as simple as asking children what things seem like to them. Sometimes, however, what they say in stories and play is even more revealing. Vivian Paley has documented her efforts to find out what the world looks like to the children in her classrooms, using their play, their stories, and what they say about those stories.[6] Carolyn Steedman recorded a group of young girls negotiating as they collaborated on a story over a period of several days.[7] Thus she had two sources of insight—their story, and their discussions as they constructed the story. And as long ago as 1959, in her classic work *The Magic Years,* Selma Fraiberg described the inner world of toddlers, using a combination of careful observation and her knowledge of mental development to put together a picture of the child's experience of life.[8] More work like this needs to be done now, in light of the vast knowledge we have acquired since Fraiberg completed her work. Teachers often need to engage in a form of imaginative role-playing in order to try and see the world from the child's perspective. Such role playing, as we know from early childhood, takes time and energy, and is not easily replaced by the shorthand of labels or undifferentiated sympathy. Teachers who make a habit of this kind of introspection often find that the question of how to guide a certain child or handle a particular situation answers itself when they begin to imagine the child's inner world. But it is not only teachers who can benefit from a different view of children.

IMPLICATIONS FOR RESEARCHERS

My focus is at odds with the emphases and approaches of many of my colleagues in developmental psychology. Yet the ideas and descriptions offered here offer ideas for how research might get a fuller, richer, and more accurate picture of young children. I do not believe that the more experimental approaches currently favored need conflict with the more interpretive and naturalistic approach supported here; instead, I think that experiments will be more useful and powerful when they are set in the context of a greater wealth of naturalistic observation. Moreover, I think that elegant and rigorous experiments may be designed to ask questions that have not been addressed fully enough in the past. Several specific recommendations are in order. The first is deceptively simple. Developmental psychologists need to spend more time making detailed observations of the children they study. This is true not only for those psychologists interested in some aspect of child development, but even for those who focus more on the development of a given process or ability such as language, memory, or problem solving. Even if the ultimate goal is precise experiments that isolate variables and make specific predictions, we need to go back and do what we rarely did: conduct a kind of naturalist's study of young children in their everyday lives. Part of what makes observations of this sort so valuable is that they capture changes that happen in real time. Often children shift back and forth between two spheres of experience, or two levels of ability in a domain, within five or ten minutes. Seeing and understanding these changes is essential to gaining a full picture of children's inner lives and the components of human development. When watching young children, whether in naturalistic settings or even in the lab, it is clear that much happens within short periods of time. A lot goes on in any experiment between the time the condition is set (the manipulation) and when the target behavior is recorded. This part of the data is valuable and should be looked at more closely. For some, such as Susan Sugarman, the sequence of behaviors that takes place within the experimental setting is the focus of investigation. We need more research like this.[9]

If one watches children over time, doing things they naturally do, the shifts, inconsistencies, and quirks almost force one to take note of the subjective—to wonder about what kinds of experience the agent of all these shifts must be having. Bruner has talked about the moment in a narrative when the author tweaks you into acknowledging that the world you temporarily inhabit (the fictive world), was created by someone.[10] If children are creating and exploring spheres of experience, their words and gestures may well serve a sort of authorial function. We need to pay close enough attention to find out if this is so.

One of the most interesting but difficult tasks for psychologists is to find ways to disentangle processes and influences so that they can begin to identify important principles of human behavior and experience. Too often, however, this drive toward isolating causes, discarding "noise," has left researchers looking at a phenomenon that has no reality or meaning in real people's lives. This is never more true than in the case of young children, who are by definition deeply tied to, if not embedded in, their context (the room, the person, the topic, the activity), and are nearly always in motion cognitively, emotionally, and physically. This means that developmental researchers need to find ways to describe, explain, and predict that take into account that often feelings, thoughts, and actions all come together in any given moment of a child's behavior. A child who cannot solve a certain cognitive task because he is too scared, or not scared enough, will give very different pictures of his cognitive ability. Allowing for this fact will entail much more than making tasks seem relevant or interesting to children—sprucing up the stimuli, using friendlier experimenters, and so forth. It will require thinking about any given cognitive domain in a new way. In her beautiful, sad book about a Hmong family and a U.S. medical team, *The Spirit Catches You and You Fall Down,* Anne Fadiman describes her interest in viewing a culture or cultures from the edges, or from the line where two cultures meet and/or miss:

> I have always felt that the action most worth watching is not at the center of things but where edges meet. I like shorelines, weather fronts, international borders. There are interesting frictions and incongruities in these places, and often, if you stand at the point of tangency, you can see both sides better than if you were in the middle of either one.[11]

The value of noticing behaviors that appear to be peripheral or unimportant can be seen in other scientific domains. The biologist Frans de Waal's first observations of primates led him to realize that many primates excel at peacemaking. He once saw two chimpanzees fighting. After a quarrel so vicious that the other chimps moved aside, the two retreated to separate branches. A few minutes later, one of them reached his hand out to the other, and within moments they were kissing. This is when de Waal took a picture. A moment that might have seemed after the fact, or extraneous to the target aggressive behavior, held the clue to a new insight about primates and became the focus of de Waal's interest—and led him to groundbreaking discoveries about what really goes on among chimpanzees.[12] This story holds a lesson for developmental psychologists.

One good way to understand children's minds, and their experience, more fully (and therefore more accurately) is to pay more attention to the shifts, the edges, the transformations, rather than the endpoints of any given situation or activity. Inevitably this will lead us to understand that most processes or skills that we want to know about can only be understood as integrating feeling, form, situation, motion, and thought. To pry these strands apart is to lose the phenomena we most want to understand.

We can begin this new approach with the premise that children are actively seeking and creating meaning in most of their everyday activities. By asking what the experience means to a child, we can create models that begin with children's experience—their inner lives—while ensuring that those models capture the mixture of feeling, thought, action, and form that seems so central to children's activities.

The wonder we feel when a child turns a car into a crocodile, or spins a tale of real mommies and magic cats, should not and need not prevent us from paying serious scientific attention to such important matters. The young child approaches her world with a mixture of seriousness and delight that is matched only by the work of the greatest artists and scientists. Before we mold her behavior into processes that seem manageable and familiar to us, we would do well to enter her mental worlds, and to watch her closely as she moves among them.

Notes

Index

Notes

1. What We See and What We Miss

1. B. Rogoff, "Sociocultural Family Resemblances and Distinctions: Participation in Sociocultural Activity or Links between Individual and Activity," paper delivered at the Society for Research in Child Development, Tampa, Fla., April 2003.
2. R. Schweder and R. Levine, eds., *Culture Theory* (Cambridge, Eng.: Cambridge University Press, 1984).
3. H. Werner, *Grundfragen der Sprachphysiognomik* (Leipzig, Ger.: Barth, 1932), translated as *Comparative Psychology of Mental Development* (New York: International Universities Press, 1973), 179–180.
4. S. Carey, "Knowledge of Number: Its Evolution and Ontogenesis," *Science* 242 (1998): 641–642; S. Carey, "Evolutionary and Ontogenetic Foundations of Arithmetic," *Mind and Language* 16, no. 1 (2001): 37–55; E. Spelke, "Core Knowledge," in *Attention and Performance,* vol. 20: *Functional Neuroimaging of Visual Cognition,* ed. N. Kanwisher and J. Duncan (Oxford, Eng.: Oxford University Press, 2003).
5. K. Chukovsky, *From Two to Five* (Berkeley: University of California Press, 1968).
6. M. Halliday, *Learning How to Mean: Explorations in the Development of Language* (New York: Elsevier, 1975).
7. D. Albright, "Literary and Psychological Modes of the Self," in *The Remembering Self,* ed. U. Neisser and R. Fivush (Cambridge, Eng.: Cambridge University Press, 1994), 19.
8. J. Piaget, "Jean Piaget Archives," from www.jeanpiaget.org (accessed 10/03/03).

9. J. Glick et al., "Piaget, Vygotsky, and Werner," in *Toward a Holistic Developmental Psychology,* ed. S. Wapner and B. Kaplan (Hillsdale, N.J.: Lawrence Erlbaum, 1985).
10. J. M. G. Itard, *The Wild Boy of Aveyron* (New York: Appleton-Century-Crofts, 1982). See also R. Shattuck, *The Forbidden Experiment: The Story of the Wild Boy of Aveyron* (New York: Kodansha International, 1980).
11. U. Neisser, *Cognition and Reality* (New York: W. H. Freeman, 1976).
12. J. H. Flavell, E. R. Flavell, and F. L. Green, "Development of the Appearance-Reality Distinction," *Cognitive Psychology* 15 (1983): 95–120; J. H. Flavell, F. L. Green, and E. R. Flavell, "Development of Knowledge about the Appearance-Reality Distinction," *Monographs of the Society for Research in Child Development* 51, no. 1 (1986); R. DeVries, "Constancy of Genetic Identity in the Years Three to Six," *Monographs of the Society for Research in Child Development* 34 (1969).
13. C. Rice et al., "When Three-Year-Olds Pass the Appearance-Reality Test," *Developmental Psychology* 33, no. 1 (1997): 54–61.
14. E. Maccoby, "Gender and Relationships: A Developmental Account," *American Psychologist* 45 (1990): 513–520.
15. J. Dore et al., "Transitional Phenomena," *Journal of Child Language* 3 (1976): 13–29.
16. D. P. Wolf and L. Kruger, "Play and Narrative in Inhibited Children: A Longitudinal Case Study," in *Children at Play: Clinical and Developmental Approaches to Meaning and Representation,* ed. A. Slade and D. P. Wolf (Oxford, Eng.: Oxford University Press, 1994).
17. S. Gaskins, "Children's Daily Activities in a Mayan Village: A Culturally Grounded Description," *Cross-Cultural Research* 34, no. 4 (2000): 375–389.
18. B. Rogoff, *The Cultural Nature of Human Development* (Oxford, Eng.: Oxford University Press, 2003).
19. M. Donaldson, *Children's Minds* (Glasgow: William Collins, 1978).
20. Z. M. Istomina, "The Development of Voluntary Memory in Preschool-age Children," *Soviet Psychology* 13 (1975): 5–64. See also S. D. Barkhatova, Z. M. Istomina, and V. I. Samokhvalova, "Age Differences in Correlation between Different Types of Memory," *Sovetskaya Pedagogika* 9 (1966): 49–57.
21. A. McCabe, "The Whole World Could Hear: The Structure of Haitian

American Children's Narratives," paper delivered at the Thirty-third Meeting of the Jean Piaget Society, Chicago, Ill., June 2003.

22. P. Miller and L. Sperry, "Early Talk about the Past: The Origins of Conversational Stories of Personal Experience," *Journal of Child Language* 15 (1988): 293–315.
23. R. Fivush and J. Hudson, eds., *Knowing and Remembering in Young Children* (Cambridge, Eng.: Cambridge University Press, 1990).
24. P. Harris, *The Work of the Imagination* (Malden, Mass.: Blackwell, 2000).
25. R. Brown, *A First Language: The Early Stages* (Cambridge, Mass.: Harvard University Press, 1973).
26. Chukovsky, *From Two to Five.*
27. C. Lewis, "Our Native Use of Words," in *Dimensions of Language Experience,* ed. C. Winsor (New York: Agathon, 1975), 143.
28. J. Sully, *Studies of Childhood* (1895; London: Free Association Books, 2000); C. Darwin, "A Biographical Sketch of an Infant," *Quarterly Review of Psychology and Philosophy* 2, no. 7 (1877): 285–294; J. Piaget, *Origins of Intelligence in the Child* (London: Routledge and Kegan Paul, 1936); Halliday, *Learning How to Mean.*
29. S. Sugarman, "The Priority of Description in Developmental Psychology," *International Journal of Behavioral Development* 10 (1987): 391–414.
30. A. Gopnik, A. Meltzoff, and P. Kuhl, *The Scientist in the Crib* (New York: HarperCollins, 1999).
31. M. Maratsos, "Grammatical Acquisition," *Handbook of Child Psychology,* ed. W. Damon (New York: John Wiley, 1998).
32. M. Franklin, personal communication, June 2003.
33. S. Sugarman, "The Cognitive Basis of Classification in Very Young Children: An Analysis of Object-Ordering Trends," *Child Development* 52, no. 4 (Dec. 1981): 1172–1178.

2. A Glance Backward

1. H. Bloom, *The Anxiety of Influence: A Theory of Poetry* (Oxford, Eng.: Oxford University Press, 1973).
2. J. J. Rousseau, *Emile; or, On Education,* trans. A. Bloom (New York: Basic Books, 1979).
3. J. M. G. Itard, *The Wild Boy of Aveyron* (New York: Appleton-Century-

Crofts, 1982). See also R. Shattuck, *The Forbidden Experiment: The Story of the Wild Boy of Aveyron* (New York: Kodansha International, 1980).

4. R. Rymer, *Genie: A Scientific Tragedy* (New York: HarperCollins, 1993).
5. S. Pepper, *World Hypotheses: A Study in Evidence* (Berkeley: University of California Press, 1942).
6. S. Mann, *Mother Land: Recent Landscapes of Georgia and Virginia* (New York: Edwynn Houk Gallery, 1997).
7. L. Malle, *Pretty Baby* (Hollywood: Paramount, 1994); V. Nabokov, *Lolita* (New York: Putnam, 1958).
8. W. Golding, *Lord of the Flies* (New York: Penguin Books, 1999); R. Hughes, *A High Wind in Jamaica* (New York: HarperCollins, 1929).
9. J. Bruner, "Tot Thought," *New York Review of Books* 47, no. 4 (Mar. 2000).
10. L. Kohlberg, "Moral Stages and Moralization: The Cognitive-Developmental Approach," in *Moral Development and Behavior: Theory, Research, and Social Issues,* ed. J. Lickona (New York: Hold, Reinhart, and Winston, 1976). See also L. Kohlberg, *The Psychology of Moral Development: The Nature and Validity of Moral Stages,* vol. 2 (New York: Harper and Row, 1984); W. Damon, ed., *Moral Development* (San Francisco: Jossey-Bass, 1978).
11. C. Zahn-Waxler and G. Kochanska, "The Origins of Guilt," in *Socio-emotional Development: The Thirty-sixth Annual Nebraska Symposium on Motivation,* ed. R. A. Thompson (Lincoln: University of Nebraska Press, 1990), 183–257; L. Kuczynski and G. Kochanska, "Development of Children's Noncompliance Strategies from Toddlerhood to Age Five," *Developmental Psychology* 26 (1990): 398–408.
12. J. DeLoache and A. Gottlieb, *A World of Babies* (Cambridge, Eng.: Cambridge University Press, 2000).
13. W. Mischel, "Metacognition and the Rules of Delay," in *Social Cognitive Development,* ed. J. H. Flavell and L. Ross (Cambridge, Eng.: Cambridge University Press, 1981); H. Mischel and W. Mischel, "The Development of Children's Knowledge and Self-Control Strategies," *Child Development* 54 (1983): 603–619; C. B. Kopp, "Self Regulation in Childhood," in *International Encyclopedia of the Social and Behavioral Sciences,* ed. N. Smelser and P. Baltes (New York: Elsevier, 2001).
14. C. B. Kopp, "Emotional Distress and Control in Young Children," in

Emotion and Its Regulation in Early Development: New Directions for Child Development, ed. N. Eisenberg and R. A. Iabes (San Francisco: Jossey-Bass, 1992), 41–56.

15. S. Freud, *Five Lectures on Psycho-Analysis,* trans. and ed. J. Strachey, with an introduction by P. Gay (New York: Norton, 1961).
16. E. Erikson, *Childhood and Society,* 2d ed. (New York: Norton, 1963).
17. J. Bowlby, *Attachment and Loss,* vol. 1: *Attachment* (New York: Basic Books, 1969); J. Bowlby, *Attachment and Loss,* vol. 2: *Separation* (New York: Basic Books, 1973).
18. H. Harlow, "Love in Infant Monkeys," *Scientific American* 200, no. 6 (1959): 68–74.
19. J. Jaffe et al., "Rhythms of Dialogue in Infancy," *Society for Research in Child Development* 66, no. 2 (2001).
20. M. D. S. Ainsworth and B. A. Wittig, "Attachment and Exploratory Behavior of One-Year-Olds in a Strange Situation," in *Determinants of Infant Behavior,* vol. 4, ed. B. M. Foss (London: Methuen, 1969). See also M. D. S. Ainsworth, S. M. Bell, and D. J. Stayton, "Individual Differences in Strange-Situation Behavior of One-Year-Olds," in *The Origins of Human Social Relations,* ed. H. R. Schaffer (New York: Academic Press, 1971).
21. M. Taylor, *Imaginary Companions and the Children Who Create Them* (Oxford, Eng.: Oxford University Press, 1999); M. Taylor and S. M. Carlson, "The Relation between Individual Differences in Fantasy and Theory of Mind," *Child Development* 68 (1997): 436–455.
22. J. Piaget, *Play, Dreams, and Imitation in Childhood* (New York: Norton, 1962), 65.
23. A. A. Milne, *Winnie the Pooh* (London: Metuchen, 1926).
24. J. Sully, *Studies of Childhood* (1895; London: Free Association Books, 2000), 24.
25. J. Piaget, *The Child's Conception of the World* (Patterson, N.J.: Littlefield Adams, 1960).
26. J. Piaget, "Comments on Mathematical Education," in *Development in Mathematical Education: Proceedings of the Second International Congress on Mathematical Education 1972,* ed. A. G. Howson (Cambridge, Eng.: Cambridge University Press, 1973).
27. J. Piaget, *Biology and Knowledge: An Essay on the Relations between*

Organic Regulations and Cognitive Processes (Chicago: University of Chicago Press, 1971).

28. C. Trevarthen, "The Foundations of Intersubjectivity: Development of Interpersonal and Cooperative Understanding in Infants," in *The Social Foundations of Language and Thought,* ed. D. Olson (New York: Norton, 1980). See also C. Trevarthen, "On the Interpersonal Origins of Self-Concept," in *The Perceived Self: Ecological and Interpersonal Sources of Self-Knowledge,* ed. U. Neisser (Cambridge, Eng.: Cambridge University Press, 1993); C. Trevarthen, "The Concept and Foundations of Infant Intersubjectivity," in *Intersubjective Communication and Emotion in Early Ontogeny,* ed. S. Braten (Cambridge, Eng.: Cambridge University Press, 1998), 15–46.
29. J. Bruner and V. Sherwood, "Early Rule Structure: The Case of Peek a Book," in *Life Sentences: Aspects of the Social Role of Language,* ed. R. Harre (New York: John Wiley, 1976).
30. M. Cole and S. Scribner, "Cross-Cultural Studies of Memory and Cognition," in *Perspectives on the Development of Memory and Cognition,* ed. R. V. Kail and J. W. Hagen (Hillsdale, N.J.: Lawrence Erlbaum, 1977).
31. D. Klahr, "My Socks Are in the Dryer," in *Children's Thinking What Develops,* ed. R. Siegler (Hillsdale, N.J.: Lawrence Erlbaum, 1983).
32. Ibid.; R. Schank, *Tell Me a Story: A New Look at Real and Artificial Memory* (New York: Scribner's, 1990); M. T. H. Chi, "Knowledge Structures and Memory Development," in *Children's Thinking: What Develops?* ed. R. S. Siegler (Hillsdale, N.J.: Lawrence Erlbaum, 1978); J. Mandler, "Representation," in *Handbook of Child Psychology,* vol. 3: *Cognitive Development,* ed. P. H. Mussen (New York: John Wiley, 1983).
33. R. Schank and R. Abelson, *Scripts, Plans, and Goals* (Hillsdale, N.J.: Lawrence Erlbaum, 1977). See also G. A. Miller, E. Galanter, and K. H. Pribram, *Plans and the Structure of Behavior* (New York: Henry Holt, 1986).
34. K. Nelson and J. Gruendel, "Children's Scripts," in *Event Representations: Structure and Function in Development,* ed. K. Nelson (Hillsdale, N.J.: Lawrence Erlbaum, 1986), 21–46.
35. J. Lucariello and K. Nelson, "Slot-Filler Categories as Memory Organizers for Young Children," *Developmental Psychology* 21 (1985): 272–282; J. Lucariello and K. Nelson, "Context Effects on Lexical Specificity in

Maternal and Child Discourse," *Journal of Child Language* 13 (1986): 507–522.

36. L. Vygotsky, *Mind in Society: The Development of Higher Psychological Processes,* ed. M. Cole (Cambridge, Mass.: Harvard University Press, 1978). See also A. Kozulin, ed. and trans., *Thought and Language* (Cambridge, Mass.: MIT Press, 1986).
37. A. Brown, "Learning, Remembering, and Understanding," in *Handbook of Child Psychology,* vol. 3: *Cognitive Development,* ed. P. H. Mussen (New York: John Wiley, 1983). See also J. H. Flavell, "Metacognition and Cognitive Monitoring: A New Area of Cognitive-Developmental Inquiry," *American Psychologist* 34 (1979): 906–911.
38. R. S. Siegler, *Emerging Minds: The Process of Change in Children's Thinking* (Oxford, Eng.: Oxford University Press, 1996).
39. D. Newman, P. Griffin, and M. Cole, "Social Constraints in Laboratory and Classroom Tasks," in *Everyday Cognition: Its Development in Social Context,* ed. B. Rogoff and J. Lave (Cambridge, Mass.: Harvard University Press, 1984).
40. M. Donaldson, *Children's Minds* (Glasgow: William Collins, 1978).
41. D. K. O'Neill, "Two-Year-Old Children's Sensitivity to a Parent's Knowledge State When Making Requests," *Child Development* 67, no. 2 (1996): 659–677.
42. R. Kavanaugh et al., "Who Is Really in Grandmother's Bed?" paper delivered at the Biennial Meeting of the Society for Research in Child Development, Minneapolis, Minn., April 2001.
43. J. Perner, S. R. Leekam, and H. Wimmer, "Three-Year-Olds' Difficulty with False Belief: The Case for a Conceptual Deficit," *British Journal of Developmental Psychology* 5, no. 2 (1987): 125–137.
44. P. Harris, *The Work of the Imagination* (Malden, Mass.: Blackwell, 2000), 195.
45. R. Kavanaugh and P. Harris, "Is There Going to Be a Real Fox in Here? The Exploration of a Shared Fantasy by Young Children," paper delivered at the Biennial Meeting of the Society for Research in Child Development, Albuquerque, N.M., April 1999.
46. I. Bretherton and M. Beeghly, "Talking about Internal States: The Acquisition of an Explicit Theory of Mind," *Developmental Psychology* 18 (1982): 906–921.

47. J. Dunn, "Family Talk about Feeling States and Children's Later Understanding of Emotions," *Developmental Psychology* 27 (1991): 448–455.
48. J. Perner, *Understanding the Representational Mind* (Cambridge, Mass.: MIT Press, 1991).
49. K. Nelson, D. Plesa, and S. Henseler, "Children's Theory of Mind: An Experiential Interpretation," *Human Development* 41 (1998): 7–29.
50. M. Franklin, "Considerations for a Psychology of Experience: Heinz Werner's Contribution," *Journal of Adult Development* 7, no. 1 (2000): 31–40.
51. N. Stein and T. Trabasso, "What's in a Story?" in *Advances in Instructional Psychology*, vol. 2, ed. R. Glasner (Hillsdale, N.J.: Lawrence Erlbaum, 1982): 213–267.

3. Spheres of Reality in Childhood

1. S. Greenfield, *Journey to the Centers of the Mind: Toward a Science of Consciousness* (New York: W. H. Freeman, 1995), 1.
2. W. L. Haight and P. Miller, *Pretending at Home: Early Development in a Sociocultural Context* (Albany: State University of New York Press, 1993); A. Slade and D. P. Wolf, eds., *Children at Play* (Oxford, Eng.: Oxford University Press, 1994); D. G. Singer and J. L. Singer, *The House of Make-Believe: Children's Play and the Developing Imagination* (Cambridge, Mass.: Harvard University Press, 1990); B. S. Smith, *The Ambiguity of Play* (Cambridge, Mass.: Harvard University Press, 1997).
3. H. Werner, *The Comparative Psychology of Mental Development* (New York: International Universities Press, 1973).
4. M. Franklin, "Considerations for a Psychology of Experience: Heinz Werner's Contribution," *Journal of Adult Development* 7, no. 1 (2000): 31–40, quotation from p. 34.
5. Alfred Schutz put forth a similar idea, terming it "provinces of meaning," in A. Schutz, *Collected Papers: The Problem of Social Reality*, vol. 1 (The Hague: Martinus Nijhoff, 1971).
6. P. Harris, *The Work of the Imagination* (Malden, Mass.: Blackwell, 2000).
7. A. Lillard, "Pretend Play as Twin Earth: A Social-Cognitive Analysis," *Developmental Review* 21 (Dec. 2001): 495–531, quotation from p. 495.
8. G. Bateson, "A Theory of Play and Fantasy," in *Steps to an Ecology of Mind* (Chicago: University of Chicago Press, 1972).

9. J. Goodnow, "Collaborative Rules: From Shares of the Work to Rights to the Story," in *Interactive Minds,* ed. P. Baltes and U. Staudinger (Cambridge, Eng.: Cambridge University Press, 1996), 163–193.
10. D. P. Wolf and H. Gardner, "Style and Sequence in Early Symbolic Play," in *Symbolic Functioning in Childhood,* ed. N. Smith and M. Franklin (Hillsdale, N.J.: Lawrence Erlbaum, 1979).
11. E. First, "The Leaving Game, or I'll Play You and You Play Me: The Emergence of Dramatic Role Play in Two-Year-Olds," in Slade and Wolf, *Children at Play,* 111–132.
12. R. Emde, D. P. Wolf, and D. Oppenheim, eds., *Revealing the Inner Worlds of Young Children: The MacArthur Story Stem Battery and Parent-Child Narratives* (Oxford, Eng.: Oxford University Press, 2003).
13. S. Greenspan and A. Lieberman, "Representational Elaboration and Differentiation: A Clinical-Quantitative Approach to the Clinical Assessment of Two- to Four-Year-Olds," in Slade and Wolf, *Children at Play,* 3–32.
14. Harris, *Work of the Imagination.*
15. J. Bruner and J. Lucariello, "Monologue as Narrative Recreation of the World," in *Narratives from the Crib,* ed. K. Nelson (Cambridge, Mass.: Harvard University Press, 1989).
16. S. Engel, *The Stories Children Tell: Making Sense of the Narratives of Childhood* (New York: W. H. Freeman, 1995).
17. S. Levin, "Concerning What Kind of Speech Act a Poem Is," in *Pragmatics of Language and Literature,* ed. T. A. van Dijk (Amsterdam: North-Holland, 1976).
18. Bruner and Lucariello, "Monologue as Narrative Recreation of the World."
19. K. Nelson, *Language in Cognitive Development: The Emergence of the Mediated Mind* (Cambridge, Eng.: Cambridge University Press, 1996); K. Nelson, *Making Sense: The Acquisition of Shared Meaning* (Orlando, Fla.: Academic Press, 1985).
20. S. Brice-Heath, *Ways with Words* (Cambridge, Eng.: Cambridge University Press, 1983).
21. Engel, *Stories Children Tell.*
22. Franklin, "Considerations for a Psychology of Experience."
23. J. Bruner, *Acts of Meaning* (Cambridge, Mass.: Harvard University Press, 1990).

24. S. Freud, "Formulations on the Two Principles of Mental Functioning," in *The Freud Reader,* ed. P. Gay (New York: Norton, 1989).
25. P. Roth, *The Facts: A Novelist's Autobiography* (New York: Farrar, Straus, and Giroux, 1988); J. Kincaid, *Autobiography of My Mother* (New York: Farrar, Straus, and Giroux, 1995).
26. A. Phillips, "The Interested Party," in *The Beast in the Nursery* (New York: Pantheon, 1998).
27. Bruner, *Acts of Meaning;* J. Bruner, *Possible Minds, Possible Worlds* (Cambridge, Mass.: Harvard University Press, 1986).
28. J. Joyce, *Ulysses* (New York: Samuel Roth, 1929); D. Defoe, *The Fortunes and Misfortunes of the Famous Moll Flanders* (New York: Heritage, 1942).
29. Roth, *The Facts.*
30. A. Luria, *Language and Cognition* (New York: Wiley, 1981).
31. M. Davol and R. Sabuda, *The Paper Dragon* (New York: Atheneum, 1997).
32. Alice McCabe, "The Whole World Could Hear: The Structure of Haitian American Children's Narratives," paper presented at the Thirty-third annual meeting of the Jean Piaget Society, Chicago, 2003.
33. J. Wooley, "Thinking about Fantasy: Are Children Fundamentally Different Thinkers and Believers from Adults?" *Child Development* 68, no. 6 (1997): 991–1011.
34. Lillard, "Pretend Play as Twin Earth."

4. Toward a More Complete Understanding of Children

1. V. Paley, *Mollie Is Three: Growing Up in School,* introduction by M. Cole (Chicago: University of Chicago Press, 1986); W. Percy, *The Message in the Bottle* (New York: Farrar, Straus, and Giroux, 1975).
2. J. Huttenlocher, S. Duffy, and S. Levine, "Infants and Toddlers Discriminate Amount: Are They Measuring?" *Psychological Science* 13, no. 3 (2002): 244–249, quotation from p. 245.
3. J. Woolley and E. Boerger, "Development of Beliefs about the Origins and Controllability of Dreams," *Developmental Psychology* 38, no. 1 (2002): 24.
4. D. Reiss et al., *The Relationship Code: Deciphering Genetic and Social Influences on Adolescent Development* (Cambridge, Mass.: Harvard University Press, 2000).

5. J. T. Bruer, *The Myth of the First Three Years: A New Understanding of Early Brain Development and Lifelong Learning* (New York: Free Press, 1999).
6. J. Brooks-Gunn, W. Han, and J. Waldfogel, "Maternal Employment and Child Cognitive Outcomes in the First Three Years of Life: The NICHD Study of Early Child Care," *Child Development* 23, no. 4 (2002): 1052–1072. Research on outcomes can of course be extremely valuable. For instance the link between risk of depression in early childhood and maternal depression has been well documented and has spurred important social programs.
7. J. Piaget, *Play, Dreams, and Imitation in Childhood* (New York: Norton, 1962).
8. J. Flavell, "Discussion of *Play, Dreams, and Imitation*," paper delivered at the Thirty-third Annual Meeting of the Jean Piaget Society, Chicago, Ill., June 2003.
9. W. James, "The Self," in *Psychology: The Briefer Course* (New York: Henry Holt, 1892), 41–49.
10. S. Koch, D. Finkelman, and F. Kessel, eds., *Psychology in Human Context* (Chicago: Chicago University Press, 1999).
11. H. Werner, *The Comparative Psychology of Mental Development* (New York: International Universities Press, 1973).
12. U. Bronfenbrenner, *The Ecology of Human Development: Experiments by Nature and Design* (Cambridge, Mass.: Harvard University Press, 1979).
13. R. Brown, *A First Language: The Early Stages* (Cambridge, Mass.: Harvard University Press, 1973).
14. U. Bronfenbrenner and J. C. Condry Jr., *Two Worlds of Childhood: U.S. and U.S.S.R.* (New York: Russell Sage Foundation, 1971).
15. P. Miller and W. Haight, *Pretending at Home: Early Development in a Sociocultural Context* (Albany: State University of New York Press, 1993).
16. M. Shatz, *A Toddler's Life: Becoming a Person* (Oxford, Eng.: Oxford University Press, 1994).
17. J. Dunn, "Naturalistic Observations of Children in Their Families," in *Researching Children's Experience*, ed. S. Greene and D. Hogan (London: Sage, 2004).
18. C. Richards and J. Sanderson, "The Role of Imagination in Facilitating Deductive Reasoning in Two-, Three-, and Four-Year-Olds," *Cognition* 72 (1999): B1–B9.

19. Piaget, *Play, Dreams, and Imitation;* L. Vygotsky, *Thought and Language,* trans. and ed. A. Kozulin (Cambridge, Mass.: MIT Press, 1986); L. Vygotsky, *Mind in Society: The Development of Higher Psychological Processes,* ed. M. Cole (Cambridge, Mass.: Harvard University Press, 1978).
20. D. Stern, *The Interpersonal World of the Human Infant* (New York: Basic Books, 1985).
21. D. Meier, *In Schools We Trust: Creating Communities of Learning in an Era of Testing and Standardization* (Boston: Beacon Press, 2002), 91.
22. E. Duckworth, *Tell Me More: Listening to Learners Explain* (New York: Teacher's College Press, 2001).
23. R. Emde, D. Wolf, and D. Oppenheim, eds., *Revealing the Inner Worlds of Young Children: The MacArthur Story Stem Battery and Parent-Child Narratives* (Oxford, Eng.: Oxford University Press, 2003).
24. C. Darwin, "A Biographical Sketch of an Infant Mind," *Quarterly Review of Psychology and Philosophy* 2, no. 7 (1877): 285–294.
25. M. Donald, *Origins of the Modern Mind: Three Stages in the Evolution of Culture and Cognition* (Cambridge, Mass.: Harvard University Press, 1991); M. Tomasello, *The Cultural Origins of Human Cognition* (Cambridge, Mass.: Harvard University Press, 2003); Vygotsky, *Thought and Language.*
26. M. Donaldson, *Human Minds: An Exploration* (New York: Allen Lane, 1993).
27. J. H. Flavell, F. L. Green, and E. R. Flavell, *Young Children's Knowledge about Thinking,* monograph of the Society for Research in Child Development 60C1, no. 243 (1995): 1–95; A. L. Brown, "The Development of Memory: Knowing, Knowing about Knowing, and Knowing How to Know," *Advances in Child Development and Behavior* 10 (1975): 103–152; and J. H. Flavell, "Metacognitive Aspects of Problem Solving," in *The Nature of Intelligence,* ed. L. B. Resnick (Hillsdale, N.J.: Lawrence Erlbaum, 1976), 231–236.
28. Vygotksy, *Thought and Language;* Vygotsky, *Mind in Society.*
29. G. Wells, *The Meaning Makers* (Portsmouth, N.H.: Heinemann, 1986).
30. J. Piaget, *The Language and Thought of the Child* (New York: Routledge and Kegan Paul, 1971), n.p.
31. K. Bartsch and H. Wellman, *Children Talk about the Mind* (Oxford, Eng.: Oxford University Press, 1995); H. Ginsburg, *Entering the Child's Mind:*

The Clinical Interview in Psychological Research and Practice (Cambridge, Eng.: Cambridge University Press, 1997).

32. C. Steedman, *Strange Dislocations: Childhood and the Idea of Human Interiority, 1780–1930* (Cambridge, Mass.: Harvard University Press, 1995).
33. M. Langendal, personal communication, April 2003.
34. J. Bruner, *Making Stories: Law, Literature, Life* (New York: Farrar, Straus, and Giroux, 2002).
35. R. Kavanaugh and P. Harris, "Is There Going to Be a Real Fox in Here? The Exploration of a Shared Fantasy by Young Children," paper delivered in a Symposium at the Biennial Meeting of the Society for Research in Child Development, Albuquerque, N.M., April 1999.
36. P. Harris, *The Work of the Imagination* (Malden, Mass.: Blackwell, 2000).
37. K. Nelson, *Language in Cognition: The Development of the Mediated Mind* (Cambridge, Eng.: Cambridge University Press, 1996).
38. James, "The Self," 41–49.
39. M. Lewis, *Shame: The Exposed Self* (New York: Free Press, 1992).
40. J. Kagan, *The Nature of the Child* (New York: Basic Books, 1984).
41. D. Wolf, personal communication, 1994.
42. M. T. H. Chi, "Knowledge Structures and Memory Development," *Children's Thinking: What Develops?* ed. R. S. Siegler (Hillsdale, N.J.: Lawrence Erlbaum, 1978). See also M. T. H. Chi and R. D. Koeske, "Network Representation of a Child's Dinosaur Knowledge," *Developmental Psychology* 19 (1983): 29–39.
43. S. Carey, "Are Children Fundamentally Different Kinds of Thinkers and Learners than Adults?" in *Thinking and Learning Skills,* vol. 2, ed. S. F. Chipman, J. W. Segal, and R. Glaser (Hillsdale, N.J.: Lawrence Erlbaum, 1985), 485–517.
44. A. Lillard, "Pretend Play as Twin Earth: A Social Cognitive Analysis," *Developmental Review* 21 (2001): 495–531.

5. Why This Matters, and to Whom

1. "Youthful Tendency Disorder," www.theonion.com (accessed on 12/27/00).
2. G. Wells, *The Meaning Makers* (Portsmouth, N.H.: Heinemann, 1986).
3. M. Donaldson, *Children's Minds* (Glasgow: William Collins, 1978), 121.

4. J. Bruner, *Actual Minds, Possible Worlds* (Cambridge, Mass.: Harvard University Press, 1986), 149.
5. J. Piaget, *Play, Dreams, and Imitation in Childhood* (New York: Norton, 1951).
6. V. Paley, *Mollie Is Three: Growing Up in School* (Chicago: University of Chicago Press, 1986).
7. C. Steedman, *The Tidy House: Little Girls Writing* (London: Virago, 1982).
8. S. Fraiberg, *The Magic Years* (New York: Scribner's, 1959).
9. J. Sully, *Studies of Childhood,* introduction by S. Sugarman (London: Free Association Books, 2000).
10. H. Melville, *Billy Budd and Other Prose Pieces,* ed. R. T. Weaver (London: Constable, 1924).
11. A. Fadiman, *The Spirit Catches You and You Fall Down: A Hmong Child, Her American Doctors, and the Collision of Two Cultures* (New York: Farrar, Straus, and Giroux, 1997), viii.
12. F. de Waal and F. Lanting, *Bonobo, The Forgotten Ape* (Berkeley: University of California Press, 1997).

Index

Abelson, Robert, 68
Abstraction, 58, 63–64, 72–73, 134
Actual Minds, Possible Worlds (Bruner), 181
Adolescents, 180
Adults, 6, 10; behavior shaped by childhood experiences, 18–19; children as small or incomplete version of, 8, 26, 45, 66, 68, 176; conversations with children, 178; fictive worlds and, 84–85; impulse-driven children and, 49; mystery of mind, 92; narratives used by, 119; pretend scenarios initiated by, 162; as shapers of children's activities, 27
Age groups, children's: developmental path and, 66–67; imaginative work and, 86; impulsive behavior and, 12–13; language and, 24–25, 39; logical sequences and, 89, 90; memory and, 73; mixed-age groups, 40; orientation toward pretense, 99–100; problem-solving and, 29; storytelling narratives and, 133, 152–153; thought process (metacognition) and, 148
Aggression, redirection of, 50
Ainsworth, Mary, 52–54
Albright, Daniel, 15
Animals, 36, 48, 164; children pretending to be, 55, 172–173; children's stories about, 110–111, 115–117; toy animals, 70
Anxiety of Influence, The (Bloom), 45
Aristotle, 45
Artificial intelligence, 65, 68, 76
Artists, children as, 93
"As if" mode, 86, 101–102, 103, 112
Attachment, early experiences of, 51–54, 180
Attunement, 144
Authority figures, 9, 52, 118
Autism, 83
Autobiographical stories, 130, 132
Aveyron, wild boy of, 18, 45–46

Babies, 36, 41; early attachment experiences, 51; global experience of world and, 99; mental life of, 141; temperament in, 166
Baldwin, James Mark, 59
Bartsch, Karen, 151
Bateson, Gregory, 101, 111
Beast in the Nursery, The (Phillips), 121–122
Beasts, children as, 45
Biology, role in development, 47, 146
Biology and Knowledge (Piaget), 62
Bloom, Harold, 45
Body, thinking and communicating with, 14, 35, 39, 58, 183, 186
Borges, Jorge Luis, 134

Bowlby, John, 51, 52, 53
Boys, gender differences and, 23–24
Brain, 140
Bretherton, Inge, 84
Bronfenbrenner, Uri, 142, 143
Brown, Ann, 73, 74, 76, 148
Brown, Roger, 34, 142
Bruer, John T., 140
Bruner, Jerome, 64, 109, 112, 121, 192; *Actual Minds, Possible Worlds,* 181; on creation of meaning, 181, 182; on internal and external landscapes, 123; *Making Stories,* 159

Carey, Susan, 12, 168
Categories, grouping into, 42, 56
Causality, 163
Chess, memory and, 67, 167
Chi, Micheline, 67, 167
Childhood, 3, 18, 85; changeable behavior in, 187–188; distorted views of, 174–176; early experiences of, 136; ethnographies of, 144; experiential aspects, 4; impulses of, 49; inner and outer worlds of, 15; language as bridge from infancy, 146; multiple spheres of, 118; neurological development in, 140; phenomenology of, 43; play as activity and orientation, 91; as time of wildness, 46; world of work and, 174
Child-rearing practices, 19, 50
Children: abused and neglected, 46–47, 51, 146; adults contrasted with, 6, 12–13, 66; appearances and reality perceived by, 20–21, 62, 157; changeable behavior of, 12–13, 16–17; as computers, 65–71; everyday-life experiences, 10, 59, 68–69, 137, 142; in everyday situations, 19; fully engaged, 186–187; gender differences, 23; "inconsistent," 187–189; interpretation of experience, 4, 27–30, 88; language and, 24–25, 34, 36, 146–152; mathematical knowledge, 21, 22; messy (dynamic) behavior of, 11–13; in Mexico, 6–7, 27; opaque behavior of, 31–32; pictures drawn by, 152–153; preexisting ideas about, 44; as psychologists, 76–88; reasons for studying, 17–19; research and, 1, 2; as scientists, 2, 36, 42, 57–65, 91; scripts formed by, 163–165; search for meaning by, 171–172, 182; as small or incomplete adults, 8, 26, 45, 66, 68, 176; socialization of, 114; social skills of, 8, 9; study of experience of, 153–159; styles of play, 26; symbol use by, 71–76; tasks performed by, 8, 12, 28, 42–43; temperaments of, 9, 166–167; thinking of, 2; wild child metaphor, 45–57. *See also* Age groups, children's; Babies; Toddlers
Children's inner lives, 1, 4, 6, 194; adult world and, 7; babies' mental lives, 141; contextual consideration of, 32; culturally shared symbols and, 72; distorted view of, 10; imagining, 190–191; language and, 36, 147; motion and change in, 92–93; play and, 93–108; poetic quality of, 13–15; research experiments and, 138; "story stems" and, 107
Children's Minds (Donaldson), 181
Children's stories. *See* Storytelling
Children Talk about the Mind (Bartsch and Wellman), 151
Child's Conception of the World, The (Piaget), 60
Chukovsky, Kornei, 13, 34
Civilization, 18, 19, 46, 55
Clinicians, 8, 9, 55, 107
Cognitive development, 8, 28, 73; cognitive schema, 19; context in variance of

cognitive skills, 30; early attachment experiences and, 52; egocentrism and, 29; interaction with others and, 64; language and, 148, 151; play and, 55–57; use of principles, 76; wild child metaphor and, 46
Cole, Michael, 64, 137
Communication, 31, 134, 160
Community, 7, 27, 164, 185
Computers, children as, 45, 65–71
Concepts, 42–43, 68, 70, 73–74, 164
Consciousness, 124, 132, 137, 171
Context, 40, 153, 158, 193
"Cookie thief" experiment, 29, 79
Counterfactuals, 82–83
Criminals, children as, 45
Cueing, by parents, 139
Cultural differences, 50, 64, 123, 143; play and, 27, 185; research and, 193; storytelling and, 131
Cultural Origins of Human Cognition, The (Tomasello), 146
Curiosity, 121–122, 150

Darwin, Charles, 36, 59, 146
Day care centers, 36, 102, 105, 187; children's use of language in, 147–148, 150; effects of on young children, 140–141
Deferred imitation, 58
Defoe, Daniel, 123
DeLoache, Judy, 50
Development, 91, 93; developmental problems, 83; linear misconception of, 177–180; neurological, 140; storytelling and, 133–134; theory of, 4; "what if" scenarios in, 113
Dickinson, Emily, 131
Donaldson, Margaret, 29, 79, 148, 181
Dramatists, 26
Dramatizations, 136
Dreams, 81
Duckworth, Eleanor, 145
Dunn, Judy, 84, 143

Education, 6, 19, 48, 140, 177–180. *See also* Schools; Teachers
Egocentrism, 78, 79
Einstein, Albert, 1
Eliot, T. S., 131
Emde, Robert, 107, 145
Emile (Rousseau), 45, 48
Emotions, 84, 91; decrease in negative emotions, 49; experience and, 34; play and, 55, 56, 106–108; pretend scenarios and, 163; problem solving and, 33, 41; self-consciousness and, 165–166; in storytelling, 121–122
Environment, role in development, 46–47, 146
Erikson, Erik, 51
Ethnographies, 137, 144
Everyday life, 37, 62, 142; fantasy and, 124; interpretation of situations, 28; language and, 39, 146; play as key feature of, 95, 102; scripts and, 68–71; storytelling and, 134; thoughts and intentions of others, 77–81
Experience: boundaries organized around, 33; children's representations of, 136; emotion and, 34; narrative in construction of, 109; order imposed upon, 15; poetic use of language and, 13–15; real and imagined domains of, 124; spheres of, 98–100, 108, 134, 189; transformation of reality and, 4
Explorers, children as, 93

Facial expressions, 144, 162
Facts, The (Roth), 124
Fadiman, Anne, 193
Faeries, children as, 45
"False belief" experiments, 80–81, 87

Fantasy, 39, 172; narrative and, 118; play and, 55; reality interwoven with, 33, 62, 99, 118, 189–190; storytelling and, 115
Faulkner, William, 131
Feeling: feeling and nonfeeling things, 36; interplay with thought, 32–35, 91
Fictive world, 33, 83, 192; boundary with actual world, 85–86, 90; integration with actual world, 102, 123–127
First, Elsa, 106
First Language, A (R. Brown), 34, 142
Fivush, Robyn, 33–34
Flavell, John, 20, 141, 148
Fox-in-box experiment, 161–162
Fraiberg, Selma, 191
Franklin, Margery, 88, 98
Freud, Anna, 49
Freud, Sigmund, 51, 81–82, 117, 121
From Two to Five (Chukovsky), 13, 34

Galton, Francis, 59
Gaskins, Suzanne, 27
Gender differences, 23–24, 25, 154
Genie (child in isolated captivity), 46–47
Gestalt figure-ground, 160
Gestures, 144, 162
Girls, gender differences and, 23–24
Glick, Joseph, 18
Goethe, Johann Wolfgang von, 154
Golding, William, 48
Goodall, Jane, 125–126
Gossip, 153
Gottlieb, Alma, 50
Gratification, delayed, 50
Greenfield, Susan, 92
Guilt, 49

Haight, Wendy, 143
Halliday, Michael, 15, 36
Harlow, Harry, 51–52, 54
Harris, Paul, 33–34, 81–88, 112, 169; on children's play, 100, 102; fox-in-box experiment and, 161, 162; on imaginary scenarios, 162; sad stories read to children, 108; *Work of the Imagination, The,* 162
High Wind in Jamaica, A (R. Hughes), 48
Homework, 177
Hudson, Judith, 33
Hughes, Martin, 29
Hughes, Richard, 48
Hypothetical situations, 84

Imagination, 82–83
Impulses, 47–51
Infancy and infants, 12, 138–139, 140, 146, 177
In Schools We Trust (Meier), 145
"Interested Party, The" (Phillips), 121–122
Interiority, 154
Istomina, Z. M., 30
Itard, Jean-Marc, 18, 45–46, 47

James, William, 141, 165
Joyce, James, 123

Kagan, Jerome, 166
Kavanaugh, Robert, 82, 161
Keller, Helen, 63
Kinkaid, Jamaica, 119
Klahr, David, 65–66, 67, 76
Knowledge, 143, 167; domains of, 12, 167–168, 170; language and, 36; level of, 35; local versus universal, 169; organized by scripts, 164; principles and, 75; social context of, 170; through action, 186
Koch, Sigmund, 142

Landscapes, internal and external, 123
Language, 10, 68–69; acquisition of, 142; first words, 63; human definition and, 146; ideational and communicative functions of, 15; imagination and, 82; invented versus borrowed forms, 127–130; inventive use of, 34, 36; opaque and transparent, 130–131; stages of acquisition, 24–25; as symbolic representation, 63; vocabulary, 23, 155; wild child metaphor and, 46
Levin, Samuel, 111–112
Lewis, Claudia, 35, 186
Li, Alice, 152
Liberia, 64
Lillard, Angeline, 100, 102, 112, 171
Lion King, The (film), 104
Little League, 7, 113
Little Red Riding Hood, 79–80
Locke, John, 46
Lolita (Nabokov), 48
Lord of the Flies (Golding), 48
Love, well-being and, 51–52
Lucariello, Joan, 70, 109
Luria, Alexander, 124

Macarthur Story Stem, 107, 145–146
Maccoby, Eleanor, 23–24, 25
Magic, 96, 97, 100, 102, 103, 134
Magic Years, The (Fraiberg), 191
Make-believe, 1, 39, 77, 99, 161–162, 171. *See also* Pretense
Making Stories (Bruner), 159
Malle, Louis, 48
Mandler, Jean, 67
Mann, Sally, 46
Maratsos, Michael, 36
Mathematics, 21–22, 23, 40, 61, 76
Maxi (boy with chocolate bar), 80–81, 84, 86–87
Maynard the cat, 20
McCabe, Alyssa, 32, 131
Meaning, 31, 36, 171, 194; in children's stories, 109, 112; literary skill and, 34; making of, 32, 55; narrative devices and, 121; time and, 40
Meier, Deborah, 145
Memory, 15, 30, 41, 67, 73, 167
Metacognition, 152, 171
Mexico, children in, 6–7, 27
Miller, Peggy, 32, 143
Milne, A. A., 58–59
Mnemonics, 74, 90
Modeling, 105
Moll Flanders (Defoe), 123
Monkeys, social attachments of, 51–52
Moral constraints, absence of, 48
Mother-child interaction, 53–54, 64, 143, 180; make-believe and, 77, 85–86; play and, 144–145; pretending and, 100–101; theory-of-mind research and, 79
Motivation, storytelling and, 153, 159
Multiword phrases, 24, 25
Myth of the First Three Years (Bruer), 140

Nabokov, Vladimir, 48
Narratives, 84, 87; canonical and noncanonical, 109; indifference to facts, 112; play and, 103; progression toward logic, 111; socialization and, 114. *See also* Storytelling
Naturalist, model of, 5, 35–43, 59–60
Nature, 48
Neisser, Ulric, 19
Nelson, Katherine, 68–70, 71, 72, 171; Maxi story experiment, 86–87; on scripts, 163, 164; on theory of mind, 88–89
Newman, Dennis, 76

Numerical reasoning, 8, 41, 75, 93
Nursery schools, 26, 153, 186

O'Neill, Daniella, 79
Origins of the Modern Mind (Donald), 146
Orphans, 51
"Our Native Use of Words" (Lewis), 35

Paley, Vivian, 191
Paper Dragon, The (Davol and Sabuda), 127
Parents, 4, 5, 114; attitudes toward learning, 177; attitudes toward play, 94; child's attachment to, 52, 54; community and, 7; cueing of children by, 139; emotional connection to, 34, 36; internalized by children, 32; perspective of, 8; scientific researchers and, 182–183
Passions, unrestrained, 46
Past, recall of the, 33
Patterners, 26
Patterns, detection of, 89–90
Peers, 8, 140, 170
Percy, Walker, 137
Perner, Joseph, 80, 81, 86
Pets, death of, 107
Phillips, Adam, 121–122
Piaget, Jacqueline, 169
Piaget, Jean, 11, 35, 42, 71, 76, 89; *Biology and Knowledge,* 62; career of, 18–19; on child as scientist, 57–58, 59–62; on children and appearances, 20; children of, 58, 169; on children's gestures and expressions, 144; *Child's Conception of the World, The,* 60; critics of, 36, 64–65, 79, 81, 167, 169, 170; on development of knowledge, 167, 170, 171, 186; as dominant figure of influence, 2–3, 45; on egocentrism, 78; on memory, 73–74; "méthode clinique" of, 151; on play, 56, 81, 83; *Play, Dreams, and Imitation in Childhood,* 141; on qualitative difference of childhood, 93; on structural changes in child's mind, 66; teachers' use of Piagetian theories, 145; three-mountain task and, 29, 151
Piaget, Laurent, 169
Piaget, Lucienne, 58, 169
Piaget on Piaget (film), 42
Pictures, 56, 136, 152–153
Planning, 146, 148
Play, 1, 23, 32, 91, 93–98, 136; boundary with work, 175; as circumscribed activity, 175; creation and crossing of boundaries, 100–102, 111; emotion as fuel for, 106–108; between fictive and actual worlds, 85; importance of, 184–186; language and, 147; logical thought and, 81–83; politics of turf and, 96; pretend scenarios, 162; skills and knowledge built through, 143; social meaning of, 37; storytelling and, 108–109, 117, 130; styles of, 26; "what if" scenarios, 103–106, 122; wild child metaphor and, 54–57
Play, Dreams, and Imitation in Childhood (Piaget), 141
Pleasure, 122, 172
Poetry, 31–32, 40, 111, 129
Prelinguistic stage, 24
Pre-operational thought, 74
Preschoolers, 78–79
Pretense, 84, 85, 91, 97, 105, 147
Pretty Baby (film), 46
Primary process thought, 81–82, 117, 118
Primates, nonhuman, 51–52, 54, 55, 89; peacemaking behavior of, 193–194; play behavior of, 101; symbolic activity and, 148

Privacy and private experience, 50, 92, 118, 122, 155
Problem solving, 8, 10, 62, 90, 146, 169; domain-specific logic and, 66, 67; emotions and, 33, 41; everyday cognition and, 37; in logic, 143–144; matching shapes, 21–22; narrated, 72; other persons' perspectives and, 79; play and, 81, 82, 95; reflectiveness and, 74
Psychologists, 2, 6, 7, 89; British, 29, 150, 176; children as, 76–88; laboratory experiments and, 21; methodologies of, 142; motives in studying children, 18; perspective of, 8; scientific method and, 137; Soviet, 30, 71; teachers and, 145. *See also* Researchers
Psychology, developmental, 1, 3, 9, 28, 72, 143; computer simulation of children's thinking, 65; "ecology of childhood," 142; experiments, 20–21, 161–162; first-person approach, 141, 160; genetic and environmental influences, 18–19; history of, 45–46; importance of, 181–183; journals of, 57; microgenetic studies, 144; naturalist model and, 36, 187, 192; role of theory in, 88–89; strands of research in, 44; study of children's experience, 153–159; theorists of, 11; third-person approach, 138

Rationality, 8, 42, 98
Reading skills, 31, 140, 178, 189
Reality: "as if" stance toward, 86, 101–102, 103, 112; fantasy and, 33, 62, 99, 118, 189–190; playfulness as orientation toward, 95; scientific experiments and, 89; spheres of, 119, 121; transformation of, 82
Recess, shortening of, 176
Reflectiveness, 72–76
Rehearsal strategy, 30
Researchers, 2, 8–9, 173, 191–194; behavior as subject of research, 136; children's play and, 26; everyday behaviors and, 20; incomplete access to children, 9; influenced by parents and teachers, 182–183; medical research compared to, 33–34. *See also* Psychologists
Rice, Catherine, 20–21, 22
Richards, Cassandra, 143
Rogoff, Barbara, 6, 7, 27, 37
Role-playing, 27, 191
Roth, Philip, 119, 124
Rousseau, Jean-Jacques, 45, 46, 47–48
Rymer, Russ, 46

Sanderson, Jennifer, 143
Schank, Roger, 67, 68
Schemas, 169
Schools, 2, 145, 176, 187. *See also* Education; Teachers
Schweder, Richard, 10
Science, 18, 36, 41, 61, 89; as Piaget's telos, 60; psychology and scientific method, 137
Scientist in the Crib, The (Gopnik et al.), 37–38
Scribner, Sylvia, 64
Scripts, in everyday life, 68–71, 76, 102, 163–165
Scripts, Plans, and Goals (Schank and Abelson), 68
Secondary process thought, 82, 117, 118
Self, development of, 141
Self-other relationship, 131–135
Sexuality, 48, 121–122, 156, 177
Shapes, matching, 21–22
Shatz, Marilyn, 143

Shyness, 166
Siblings, 7, 8, 84, 95, 108, 170; birth of, 107; rivalry with, 119–120, 121
Siegler, Robert, 74–76, 81
Simon, Herb, 65
Socialization, 114, 140
Soviet Union, 71, 143
Spelke, Elizabeth, 12
Spencer, Herbert, 59
Spirit Catches You and You Fall Down, The (Fadiman), 193
Spontaneity, 40
Steedman, Carolyn, 154, 191
Stein, Nancy, 89
Stern, Dan, 144
Storytelling, 1, 2, 23, 31, 89, 108–109; age-group differences in, 152–153; classroom (mis)use of, 178–179; contrasting themes in, 122–135; emotional content of, 107; internal and external landscapes in, 123; invented versus borrowed forms, 127–130; language play and, 130–131; literary analysis of, 32; lived versus imagined worlds, 123–127; logical sequence and, 89; self versus other in, 131–135; spheres of experience within, 109–115; sympathetic response elicited from, 32–33; wild side of, 115–122. *See also* Narratives
"Strange situation" paradigm, 53
Studies of Childhood (Sully), 36, 59
Sugarman, Susan, 36–37, 42–43
Sully, James, 36, 59–60
Syllogisms, 143
Symbols, 26, 63, 82, 90; from biology to culture, 146; children's social use of, 71–76; imagination and, 83; referents merged with, 99; as second world, 124
Syntax, 25
Taylor, Marjorie, 56
Teachers, 4, 5, 7, 56, 114, 173; attitudes toward learning, 177, 178–179; child's egocentrism and, 78–79; fully engaged child and, 186–187; perspective of, 8; psychologists and, 145, 182. *See also* Education; Schools
Tell Me More (Duckworth), 145
Temperament, 9, 166
Theory-of-mind research, 9, 79, 81, 83, 84, 87–88
Third-person approach, 138
Thought: interplay with feeling, 32–35, 91; magical, 134; nonrational, 10; primary and secondary processes, 81–82, 117–118; representational, 58; thoughts and intentions of others, 77–81
Thought and Language (Vygotsky), 146
Three-mountain task, 29, 79, 173
Time: experience evolving through, 39–40; imagination and, 82; past events recalled, 33; routines of everyday life and, 69; stories about the past, 23; storytelling and, 122, 125
"Time-outs," 183
Toddlers, 34, 36, 49, 140; attachment to mother, 53, 180; egocentric view of, 78–79; first words of, 63; grouping things into categories by, 42–43; language and, 147–148; storytelling and, 109; syllogisms solved by, 143
Tools, 72
Toys, 26, 39, 57, 102, 103–104, 173
Trabasso, Tom, 89
Transformation, play and, 97, 194
Transitional phenomena, 25
Trevarthen, Colwyn, 64
"Twin Earth," world of pretend as, 100
Two Worlds of Childhood (Bronfenbrenner), 142

Ulysses (Joyce), 123
Understanding, stages of, 76
United States, children in, 27, 143

Video data, 144, 145, 161
Violence, 48, 106
Vygotsky, Lev, 11, 56, 86, 144; on children's social use of symbols, 71–72; on language, 150; *Thought and Language*, 146

Waal, Frans de, 193–194
Wellman, Henry, 86, 151
Wells, Gordon, 150, 178
Werner, Heinz, 11, 98–99, 124, 142
Wild child, metaphor of, 45–47, 77, 91; absorption in play, 54–57; attachment to others, 51–54; impulse and, 47–51
Wilhelm Meister's Apprenticeship (Goethe), 154
Winnie the Pooh (Milne), 58–59
Wolf, Dennie, 26, 105, 166
Words, 24, 25, 72, 124
Work, 173, 174; boundary with play, 175; imaginative, 82, 86; relation to play, 94–95, 185; social meaning of, 37
Work of the Imagination, The (Harris), 162